THE **RHEUMATOID ARTHRITIS** COOKBOOK

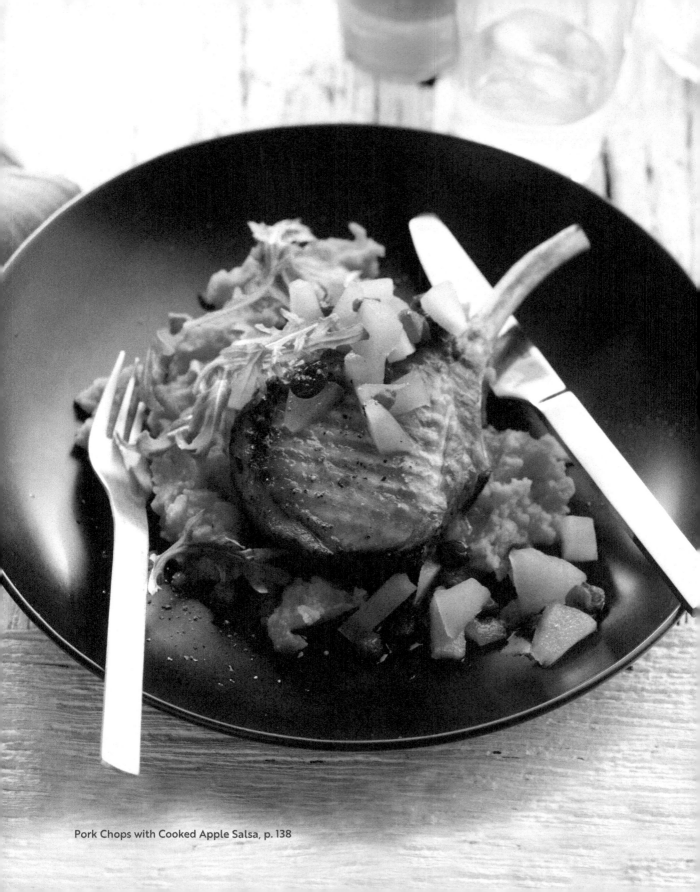

Pork Chops with Cooked Apple Salsa, p. 138

THE
RHEUMATOID
ARTHRITIS
COOKBOOK

Anti-Inflammatory Recipes to Fight Flares & Fatigue

CAITLIN SAMSON, MSACN
Clinical Nutritionist

Foreword by Kate Hope, MS, CNS

ROCKRIDGE
PRESS

This book is dedicated to you—the rheumatoid arthritis sufferer who is tired of letting this condition control your life and ready to take a natural, healing approach.

For general information on our other products and services or to obtain technical support, please contact our Customer Care Department within the United States (866) 744-2665, or outside the United States at (510) 253-0500.

Rockridge Press publishes its books in a variety of electronic and print formats. Some content that appears in print may not be available in electronic books, and vice versa.

TRADEMARKS: Rockridge Press and the Rockridge Press logo are trademarks or registered trademarks of Callisto Media Inc. and/or its affiliates, in the United States and other countries, and may not be used without written permission. All other trademarks are the property of their respective owners. Rockridge Press is not associated with any product or vendor mentioned in this book.

Cover Photography © Stocksy/Darren Muir

Photography © Stockfood/People Pictures, p.2; timo8/Shutterstock.com, p.5; Stockfood/Valerie Janssen, p.6; Merc67/Shutterstock.com, p.8; Yuliya Gontar/Shutterstock.com, p.8; Stockfood/Tina Bumann, p.12; Anukool Manoton/Shutterstock.com, p.18; Stocksy/Rowena Naylor, p.21; Stockfood/Jo Kirchherr, p.32; Stockfood/Gräfe & Unzer Verlag/mona binner PHOTOGRAPHIE, p.48; Stockfood/Victoria Firmston, p.60; Stockfood/Elle Brooks, p.74; Stockfood/Great Stock!, p.90; Stockfood/The Stepford Husband, p.102; Stockfood/Harry Bischof, p.114; Stockfood/Will Shaddock Photography, p.128; Stockfood/Keller & Keller Photography, p.146; Stockfood/Portland Photography, p.160

Backcover Photography © StockFood/Will Shaddock Photography; © StockFood/Jo Kirchherr; © StockFood/Tina Bumann

ISBN: Print 978-1-62315-863-7
eBook 978-1-62315-864-4

NATURE'S MEDICINE

Herbs and spices do so much more than flavor food. They have incredible anti-inflammatory benefits to help with autoimmune conditions, such as rheumatoid arthritis. Many herbs and spices have a long history of helping manage health conditions. Here are five of my favorites used in recipes throughout this book:

GINGER is an anti-inflammatory power-house! It inhibits the enzymes involved in the pro-inflammatory pathways and has been shown to have the same pharmacological effects as non-steroidal anti-inflammatory drugs (NSAIDs), such as aspirin and ibuprofen, without the negative side effects.

TURMERIC is an amazing spice that contains curcumin, a powerful natural chemical that helps decrease inflammation by inhibiting the enzymes of the pro-inflammatory pathways.

CINNAMON is a warm flavor that adds a nice sweet spice to food. It not only tastes great, but also helps reduce inflammation and manage blood sugar. You find this spice used in several recipes in this book.

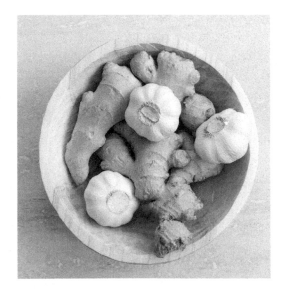

CLOVES have one of the highest antioxidant levels of any spice. You don't need to use a lot to add good flavor to your food. I love grinding them fresh in a coffee grinder before adding to a recipe. The aroma is wonderful!

GARLIC has an incredible history and is used in many cultures all over the world. It has anti-inflammatory properties, is great for heart health, and supports the immune system to ward off pathogens such as viruses, bacteria, and parasites. You will find it used in many recipes in this book for its wonderful flavor and health benefits.

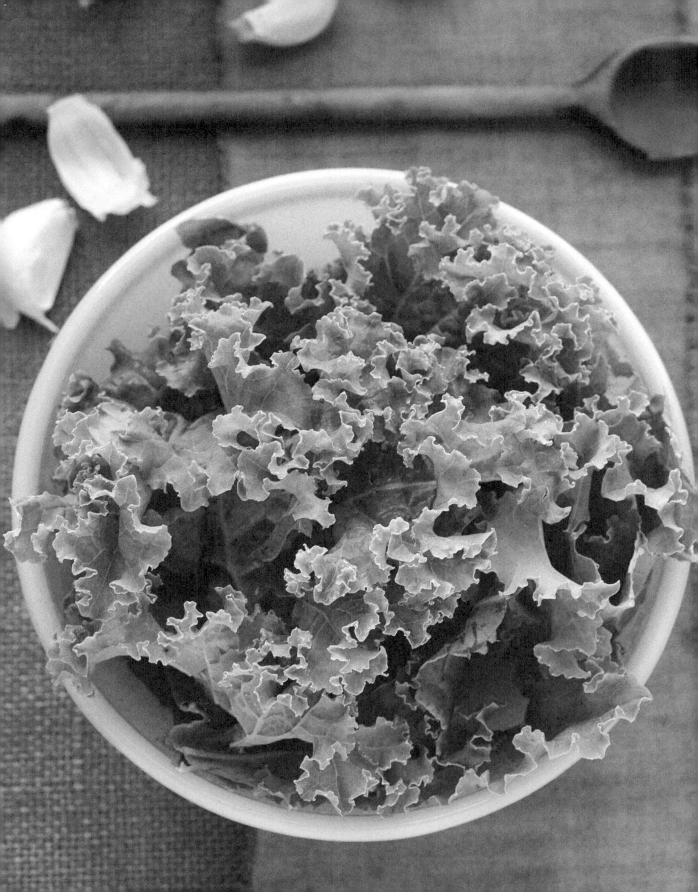

CONTENTS

FOREWORD

"The natural healing force within each of us is the greatest force in getting well."
—Hippocrates

Oftentimes, people who go into the wellness or coaching fields are motivated to help others because of the difficult health issues they themselves have had to overcome. This was the case with both Caitlin Samson and myself. We met in graduate school where we were each pursuing our master's degree in clinical nutrition. Caitlin had successfully reversed her rheumatoid arthritis (RA) and I had made great strides in my own battle with Lyme Disease. I was immediately drawn to Caitlin's sense of fortitude as someone who had not only conquered a chronic illness, but also used that struggle to fuel her way through a career in health and wellness. In fact, armed with her blended expertise in both nutrition and personal training—and a whole lot of heart—she has even competed as an accomplished marathoner! As we compared notes, we came to the conclusion that we had tapped into the healing force within ourselves, and realized that food had played a tremendous part in our individual recoveries. Now we love sharing the message that Hippocrates proclaimed more than two thousand years ago: food is medicine.

If you are one of the 1.3 million people in the United States who suffers from rheumatoid arthritis, you are all too familiar with joint pain, fatigue, and even depression. You may have already tried, or are currently trying, conventional anti-inflammatory medications such as NSAIDs, DMARDs, and steroids. Perhaps these medicines are not delivering the results you hoped for. More important, they could even be robbing your body of the necessary vitamins and minerals it needs in order to thrive.

As a Certified Nutrition Specialist, I am amazed that food as medicine is still so underrated in the medical community. I often hear stories from my clients about the many doctors who do not value the integral role food plays in mending our bodies. Did you know that ginger can have the same anti-inflammatory power as ibuprofen or aspirin? Did you know that the vitamin C in fruit helps repair joints and build collagen? Did you know that an anti-inflammatory diet full of colorful vegetables can reduce the ravages of chronic disease? You will learn these facts and more in *The Rheumatoid Arthritis Cookbook*. As Caitlin teaches you in this book, you truly are what you eat. She skillfully guides you to improved health with her all-encompassing program that includes valuable, researched information on RA; easy-to-follow meal plans; and delicious, wholesome recipes that will keep you nourished and satisfied.

I love the "Anti-Inflammatory Diet at a Glance" section on page 26. It is an easy,

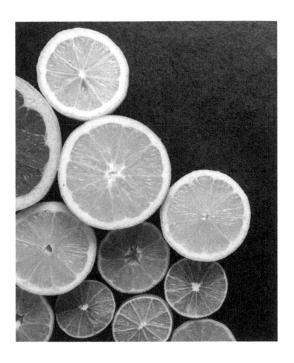
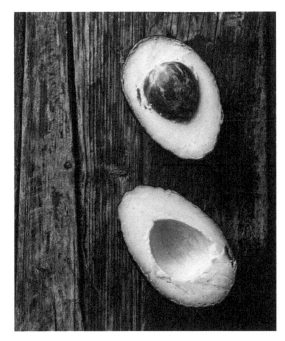

go-to guide on what to include and what to avoid when following Caitlin's wellness plan. "The RA Pantry" on page 29 is a convenient list of essential items to have on hand, including therapeutic herbs and spices. On page 28 she even offers you practical tips for easier home cooking.

Rather than continue to sift through the sea of information out there, allow Caitlin to be your nutritional guide; there is no one better to help you reclaim your health. In treating yourself to her tasty recipes (how good does a Chocolate-Avocado Smoothie or a batch of Golden Coconut Pancakes sound for breakfast?), I am confident you will find yourself on the road to recovery. So make yourself cozy with a cup of your favorite herbal tea, put your feet up, and start reading. You too will see that the answer to your suffering is not in your medicine cabinet, but has been in your kitchen all along.

Best wishes as you tap into your own healing force!

Kate Hope, MS, CNS

INTRODUCTION

Are you sick and tired of being sick and tired?

If your answer is yes, you've come to the right place. *The Rheumatoid Arthritis Cookbook* outlines how I healed my rheumatoid arthritis (RA) and other health issues through proper nutrition—and the good news is that you can too. This book is for those who feel the frustration I did about not getting appropriate nutritional guidance to help heal their condition. I wish I had known sooner how important nutrition is to our health and had simple recipes, like those included here, to help me through my journey.

My health issues go back to when I was five years old—with joint pain in my hands and feet. I realized years later that I had an autoimmune condition, RA, where my joints were mistakenly attacked because of a faulty immune system response in my body. At the time, I guess I thought this pain was normal. I am here to tell you it was *not*.

At 16, I had my gallbladder removed and felt so much better after the removal. But years later, I realized this was just a temporary fix. No one questioned *why* this happened to someone so young.

Fast-forward eight years: I suffered again from digestive issues, and I still had the RA pain but attributed this to the running I was doing. I was also tired all the time no matter how much I slept.

The final straw came some years later when I did not get my menstrual cycle for more than a year. I went back to the doctor, who said I was probably running too much. This did not make sense—I had been running this much for several years. I had the intuition that something was just not right inside my body.

I was at a loss about what to do until my sister told me about a natural health practitioner helping her. I trusted my sister and was ready to try anything to feel better. This practitioner was the only one who took a good look at my diet. His suggestions, which I followed, included whole food supplementation to help my body gently detoxify. We made several additional modifications, such as removing white sugar, refined grains, and pasteurized dairy from my diet. He slowly transitioned me into an anti-inflammatory diet to reduce inflammation and support my immune system naturally. I told myself, "If this works, I will physically see the benefit with my menstrual cycle coming back." Would you believe that in eight weeks it did?!

What was amazing about this transition was that I saw my health improve in more ways than I imagined—no more digestive issues, no more anxiety, no more fatigue, and no more RA joint pain! All of these are managed now by my lifestyle choices, not medications. My RA symptoms return only if I venture away from my healthy diet.

This experience sparked a fire in me to learn more about the science of nutrition and how it can help us heal, including the strong relationship between diet and RA. I went back to school for my master's degree in Applied Clinical Nutrition, and now I help others get their health and their lives back. I work with people who have autoimmune conditions such as RA, as well as chronic Lyme disease, anxiety, depression, chronic fatigue, ADHD, digestive issues, and hormonal imbalances. This book provides much of the information I share with my clients, and the easy-to-follow recipes use only ingredients that support your immune system and provide excellent nutritional value.

Throughout my healing journey I have learned that our bodies want to heal but we must remove the interferences. The food we eat is one thing we can control to reduce the toxic load we are exposed to. There are many other factors to consider throughout the healing process, such as the chemicals we are exposed to in our homes and the water we drink.

We also cannot forget the importance of stress management and getting enough sleep, which is the time our bodies heal. In my experience as a nutritionist and personal trainer, I have seen how important positive thinking is. So remember this is a journey. Don't get sucked into the downward spiral of negative thoughts. Be patient and excited for your new healthy life! Forgiveness and spiritual wellness are key components as well. We need to forgive ourselves and others. We need to find our purpose and meaning in life.

Following the guidelines and recipes in this book, you will experience less pain and inflammation, less fatigue and more energy, improved mental health (less anxiety and depression), and a better overall quality of life. You have the power to take action to help heal your RA symptoms. Changing your diet requires work, but it is an exciting journey, not a hardship. There are foods you should avoid but also plenty of new foods to fill your plate. Challenges will arise, but that is how we learn and grow. Remember, no one is perfect. Stay positive and enjoy the ride. You are about to embark on a life-changing journey.

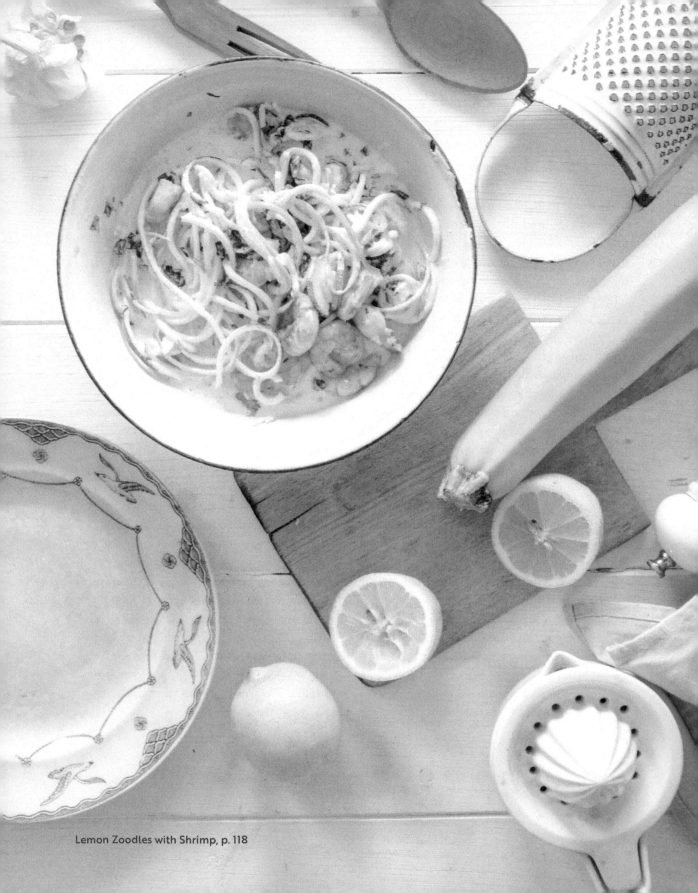

Lemon Zoodles with Shrimp, p. 118

1

RHEUMATOID ARTHRITIS & DIET

Living with rheumatoid arthritis can be frustrating and debilitating—and while some practitioners say nutrition has nothing to do with it, we know the food we eat can help reduce inflammation or exacerbate it. This chapter covers the connection between diet and RA—and nutrition's key role in healing—and empowers you to make changes to improve your health.

Empowered Eating

In today's world we are exposed to many toxins—from the air we breathe to the water we drink. While we cannot control many of these, thankfully we can control what we put in our mouths. You have the choice to eat food that either nourishes your body or harms it.

Throughout my healing experience I learned about the powerful role nutrition plays in our health. I used to think the equation was as simple as "calories in, calories out." JJ Virgin said it well: "Our bodies are not bank accounts; our bodies are chemistry labs and we need to look at diet, exercise, sleep, stress, toxicity, hormones, and digestive function." In other words, what you eat affects the functioning of every cell in your body. This just makes sense, doesn't it?

While proper nutrition may not erase every symptom of RA, it absolutely can help. Some foods exacerbate inflammation and others do not. Not sure what these are? No worries; this book covers several anti-inflammatory foods to make it easy to understand which foods could be beneficial in your diet to improve your overall well-being and reduce symptoms associated with RA such as pain and fatigue.

Nutrition can be an overwhelming topic for some. I like to keep things simple: Eat real food—one-ingredient foods. Look at food for more than its caloric value; look at the nutrients it provides for your body. I'm here to help. This book provides easy, anti-inflammatory, nutrient-dense recipes

that are great for helping people with RA. And I promise you, your taste buds will be happy too!

What Is Rheumatoid Arthritis?

RA is a chronic inflammatory disease of the joints. It is an autoimmune condition, meaning an abnormal response of the immune system is occurring. Simply put, it is as if the body is attacking its own healthy tissue. This is a painful condition that affects multiple joints—particularly the fingers, wrists, knees, and feet—and can lead to joint and bone destruction.

While many think RA is a condition that only affects older individuals, this is not always the case. It can begin at any age. In my case, I started to have RA symptoms at about five years old. And, according to the Centers for Disease Control (CDC), women are two to three times more likely to develop RA than men, and the prevalence among women may be increasing.

With RA, and all autoimmune diseases, the main goal is to support the immune system by reducing the inflammatory response. In fact, most chronic diseases (e.g., diabetes, high blood pressure, high cholesterol) are linked to inflammation, and nutrition is one major means of reducing it. I have seen many people progress nicely when they reduce inflammatory foods in their diet and introduce anti-inflammatory ones. I am excited to share information about those foods with you.

While nutrition is a major component in reducing inflammation, we must consider the whole person—body, mind, and spirit—so it is also important to look at other areas that can affect inflammation such as sleep, managing stress, exercise, and thoughts and emotions.

What Causes Rheumatoid Arthritis?

While the exact cause of RA is not known, scientific evidence points to a number of risk factors, only 30 percent of which are genetic, meaning the rest are things such as the environment and infections that lead to the development or progression of the disease. RA can result from the interaction between genetics and the various environmental factors. In other words, if RA runs in your family, you are not doomed to develop it. While you may be genetically predisposed to RA, the environment plays a significant role in altering our genes to either turn them "on" or "off."

For instance, studies have shown that smoking has a strong association with susceptibility to RA, and the standard American diet (SAD), composed of high sugar, high salt, unhealthy fats, and an excess of processed foods, has also been shown to be associated with autoimmune disease. These are factors we can control; we can stop smoking and improve our diet to reduce the inflammatory stressors we are exposed to and lessen our risk of developing RA.

With RA occurring two to three times more frequently in women than men, it is thought there is a link between hormones and the risk of developing RA. Those who have PCOS (polycystic ovarian syndrome), as well as those with irregular menstrual cycles (which may result from PCOS), have an increased risk of developing RA. The good news: if you have irregular menstrual cycles or PCOS, nutrition is a great way to help.

How Rheumatoid Arthritis Affects the Body and Mind

What makes RA challenging to live with is that it is a systemic and chronic illness affecting multiple body parts. This is something we have to manage every day, and you may not know what the next day will bring in terms of fatigue or flares. Living in pain and with constant fatigue can affect us emotionally; it is easy to feel frustration, despair, and anxiety due to our physical condition.

As for physical health, studies show that those with RA are 40 percent more likely to report fair or poor general health and 30 percent more likely to need help with personal care than those without arthritis. RA can also have a significant negative impact on work life as those with RA are more likely to change occupations, lose their jobs, be unable to find a job, and retire early compared to those without arthritis.

FLARES

Flares and fatigue can affect work performance. I remember being at work and feeling so tired. It did not matter how much I slept. The pain in my feet, hands, knees, elbows, and ankles was unbearable at times, but I had to carry on. It scares me to think where I would be now if I continued down that path. I know I would not be functioning in society as I am today.

FATIGUE

The fatigue and pain experienced with RA can also contribute to weight difficulties. Some people with RA have trouble gaining or losing weight. The inflammatory molecules that are increased in RA can accelerate muscle loss, thus leading to an increase in fat mass. An increase in fat mass can further increase inflammation in the body. Fat is not just there in our bodies doing nothing; it has

Learning to Like Your Body

To establish the right mind-set for this healing journey, start by loving yourself and liking your body. I know, not easy. It is normal to feel all sorts of emotions when you have a chronic health condition. Recognize how you feel and commit to changing it.

STAY POSITIVE Every day. Tell yourself you *can* do this. The people who have the best success are those who *believe* they can get well and *want* to get well.

BELIEVE Have faith in your body's ability to get well. It can be hard to love a body that you feel has betrayed you. However, remember our bodies are designed to heal. We must support them and remove what's interfering with the healing process.

LOVE YOURSELF When we look in the mirror, we may criticize ourselves for our weight, how big our hips are, or any number of perceived flaws. We must learn to love ourselves and see the beauty we possess on the outside and inside. Taking steps to heal involves loving ourselves enough to want to make a change.

HEAL EMOTIONAL TRAUMAS Let's face it: We all have *something* to work on from our past. Forgive yourself, and others, to open the path to healing. This emotional piece is the key to unlocking the door to optimal health.

FIND THE BLESSING It is easy to look at life and get angry and frustrated. I sometimes feel angry at my past medical practitioners for dismissing my symptoms and not exploring the root cause of my issue. However, it was really a blessing. I can truly relate to how others feel—their pain—and help them feel better.

been shown to be strongly associated with an inflammatory marker called C-reactive protein. Therefore, the more fat we have, the more inflammation we have in our bodies. For your convenience, at the end of this book there are two one-week meal plans composed of recipes from this book to help support your weight goal (page 161).

WEIGHT GAIN AND DEPRESSION

Weight gain can lead to more anxiety and despair, aggravating the vicious inflammatory cycle. Weight issues or not, depression has been shown to be higher in those with RA than the general population and can lead to poorer outcomes, including increased pain, poor sleep quality, increased risk of developing other diseases or disorders in addition to RA, and increased mortality, according to a study published in the *International Journal of Clinical Rheumatology*. Suffering from the disease can lead to an array of emotional responses. The whole-body inflammation experienced with RA can be a cause or contributor to depression, and depression is associated with inflammation.

Hang in there. There is hope—and help—to stop this cycle. By taking control of what you can, you will reduce your RA symptoms. Let's get started!

The Diet Connection

Managing RA requires a multipronged approach that includes proper nutrition, exercise, stress management, good-quality sleep—and medications for some. This book emphasizes diet because food is an integral part of our daily lives. We confront food choices several times a day. If we ignore this key piece, it will be difficult to feel well no matter what other efforts we make.

A few key nutrients play especially important roles in an anti-inflammatory diet.

- *Healthy fats,* including omega-3 fatty acids, have been shown to reduce inflammation and are associated with a lower incidence of depression.
- *Antioxidants,* found in vegetables and fruits, inhibit cell damage and protect against inflammation and the development of RA.
- *Water* is an essential part of life with a number of functions in the body. It allows us to get rid of waste products via our kidneys and is a key component in the fluid that lubricates our joints. On average, water makes up 60 percent of our body weight. We need proper hydration to function well. Even mild dehydration can lead to fatigue and a reduction in physical and mental performance. With RA, focus on hydration to support joint health and energy.
- *Vitamins* also have important antioxidant roles. Vitamin C helps repair joints and builds collagen. Vitamin E helps increase production of the body's building blocks: cartilage. Vitamin D, the "sunshine vitamin," can help suppress the autoimmune response and may help with mood disorders such as depression. Vitamin D is known to improve bone health and decrease the risk of heart disease and

The Medicine–Diet Relationship

While medications do not cure RA, they can help control it, but also produce side effects due to the nutrient depletions they create.

DMARDS (disease-modifying antirheumatic drugs) such as Methotrexate suppress the immune system. This type of drug is structurally similar to the vitamin folic acid and can interfere with its ability to reproduce cells, resulting in cell death. Its side effects include kidney failure, reddening of the skin, and gingivitis. This drug depletes or interferes with the activity of folic acid, calcium, vitamin B_{12}, and beta-carotene (a precursor to vitamin A that gives a red-orange pigment to fruits and vegetables).

NSAIDS (nonsteroidal anti-inflammatory drugs) such as ibuprofen are commonly used to reduce pain and inflammation. Their side effects include headache, rash, fluid retention, and nervousness. This medication can also deplete you of folic acid.

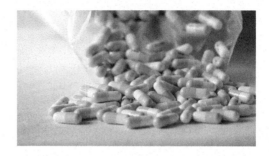

CORTICOSTEROIDS such as prednisone reduce pain and inflammation. Their side effects include insomnia, increased appetite, indigestion, and nervousness. The nutrients robbed by this medication include folic acid; vitamins A, B_6, C, D, and K; calcium; magnesium; potassium; selenium; and zinc.

It is not uncommon for someone to take one medication only to need another for the side effect that is actually caused by the nutrient depletion from the medication. I cannot overstate how important nutrients are to the proper functioning of our bodies. For instance, vitamin A helps maintain skin and bone health and supports our immune system's functioning. Vitamin B_{12} helps transmit the signals between our brain and nerves.

The following tips will help make up for the nutrient depletions from the medications noted previously:

EAT YOUR GREENS! Leafy greens are packed with nutrition, including folate (the natural form of folic acid).

EAT FEWER PROCESSED FOODS AND MORE WHOLE FOODS. Whole foods are loaded with nutrition, supplying our bodies with the nutrients needed to carry out all their processes.

BE A DETECTIVE! Read the ingredients list. We get so caught up in calories that we forget to look at what *is* in our food. Keep an eye out for these culprits: added color, canola oil, cornstarch, dextrose (a form of sugar), enriched flour, and sugar. These ingredients can exacerbate RA.

CONSIDER SUPPLEMENTATION. Even with a healthy diet, we may not reach sufficient levels of certain nutrients to replace what we lose from medications. Consider a functional/clinical nutritionist or functional medicine practitioner to help you determine the supplementation you need.

For natural sources of replenishing nutrients depleted by RA medications, include the following in your diet:

- *Calcium:* green vegetables, oranges, salmon, whole milk, yogurt
- *Folate:* beets, green vegetables (asparagus, broccoli, spinach), lentils
- *Magnesium:* lentils, nuts and seeds (sunflower seeds, almonds, walnuts), spinach
- *Potassium:* beef, chicken, fish, fruits, lentils, nuts, vegetables
- *Selenium:* beef, calves' liver, cod, pork, salmon, sardines
- *Vitamin A:* apricots, beef liver, carrots, cod liver oil, eggs, spinach, sweet potato
- *Vitamin B_6:* banana, calves' liver, lentils, spinach, trout
- *Vitamin B_{12}:* fish, meat
- *Vitamin C:* fruits (grapefruit, oranges, strawberries), vegetables (broccoli, cauliflower)
- *Vitamin D:* butter, calves' liver, eggs, salmon, tuna
- *Vitamin K:* beef liver, butter, eggs, green vegetables (broccoli, green cabbage, spinach)
- *Zinc:* lentils, liver, meat (beef, veal, chicken), oysters

certain types of cancer. Very few foods contain vitamin D. Food sources include oily fish (salmon, mackerel, herring), cod liver oil, and fortified products, including milk, juice, yogurts, and cheeses.

- *Minerals!* The processed foods that make up a large part of the standard American diet lack minerals and contain additives and preservatives that can harm our bodies. Even a primarily whole foods–based diet can lack minerals: modern-day farming practices have demineralized the soil that plants grow in, and plants receive nutrition from the soil. As a result, most of us can benefit from a whole food mineral supplement, which are foods in their whole state put into a concentrated form. These are available through health care practitioners who can determine which is best for you. If you buy supplements over the counter, be sure they are made from whole foods.

Following an Anti-Inflammatory Diet

Inflammation is not necessarily a bad thing. Acute inflammation is your body's way to repair and heal damaged tissues. However, inflammation is a tightly regulated process and, if it gets out of control, can be harmful and damaging to healthy tissues. Inflammation should be temporary not permanent. Reducing inflammation in the body is a key piece to managing RA. We can do this by adopting an anti-inflammatory diet.

Here are six guidelines for an anti-inflammatory diet:

- *Load your plate with nutritious, anti-inflammatory foods.* These include one-ingredient whole foods such as fruits, vegetables, and healthy fats like those found in avocados and fish.
- *Avoid processed and packaged foods.* Most processed items lack nutritional value and contain additives, food dyes, and preservatives that can do more harm than good, including increasing inflammation.
- *Avoid trans fat.* This chemically altered fat is associated with inflammation. It can be found in baked goods such as cookies, cakes, and muffins, as well as packaged foods such as crackers.
- *Avoid added sugar.* This does not include natural sugars such as those in fruit. Check the ingredients list on any packaged foods to see if sugar is listed; it is in many products including so-called "healthy" items like soups, breads, granola bars, and yogurts. The American Heart Association recommends limiting added sugar consumption to 25 grams (6 teaspoons) per day for women and 35 grams (9 teaspoons) per day for men.
- *Avoid artificial sweeteners.* While these are allowed in the food supply, it's important to know that some animal studies show artificial sweeteners have led to tumor development. Natural sweeteners (pure maple syrup, raw honey, stevia) are preferable to artificial ones when sweetening is needed.

Fermented Foods and Inflammation

Would you believe the pain in your joints could be from a problem in your gut? Our gastrointestinal tract houses 70 percent of our immune system! Poor gut health can contribute to the onset of RA or its severity. A healthy gut plays a critical role in maintaining immune system balance. Dysbiosis, an overgrowth of "bad" bacteria in the small intestine, can be present in RA patients due to environmental factors (poor diet) and infections. This unfavorable imbalance of bacteria leads to a "leaky gut" where the lining of the small intestine becomes hyperpermeable, letting substances pass into the bloodstream that should not. The immune system sees these particles as foreigners and mounts an attack against them, aggravating the autoimmune response.

Restoring gut health and reducing inflammation through a healthy diet that incorporates probiotics and prebiotics can help. Probiotics contribute to microbial balance and prevent the overgrowth of harmful bacteria in the gut.

Fermented foods, which are packed with probiotics (good bacteria), are beneficial to include in the diet. These foods are good sources:

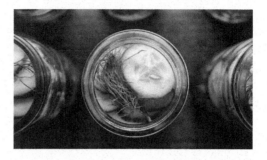

- Kefir
- Kimchi
- Kombucha
- Pickles
- Sauerkraut
- Yogurt

Keep in mind that many commercial yogurts are pasteurized or sterilized *after* they are cultured, which causes them to lose many of the good bacteria. Since many people with RA do well to avoid dairy, I recommend not consuming cow's milk yogurt (especially the flavored ones with added sugar) or kefir. Coconut kefir (which is dairy-free) is a great alternative.

Prebiotics, food for the probiotics, are also important to include in your diet. These high-fiber foods are fermented by our gut's bacteria. Here are some examples of prebiotic foods:

- Artichokes
- Dandelion greens
- Onions
- Raw garlic

- *Avoid food sensitivities.* Many of us eat foods daily that inflame our bodies! Food sensitivities are not full-blown allergies that could lead to an anaphylactic response such as hives or trouble breathing. They are hidden and have a delayed response, so they can be tricky to identify. It could be 24 to 72 hours before you experience a symptom (fatigue, headache, joint pain) related to a food sensitivity. Remove any potential offending foods for a period of time to see how you feel. Consider reintroducing these foods to see what happens. This simple test will help you see how foods affect you.

Foods that Fight Inflammation

With each bite of food, we can either add to or reduce inflammation. Anti-inflammatory foods containing powerful anti-inflammatory compounds include healthy fats, good-quality meats and fish, fruits and vegetables, and herbs and spices.

HEALTHY FATS

Anti-inflammatory omega-3 fats are found in fish, meat, and eggs from animals that are grass fed or pasture raised. These fats play a major role in preventing heart disease, the buildup of plaque in the arteries (atherosclerosis), cancer, and depression.

Additionally, at least 3 grams of fish oil per day has been shown to significantly reduce morning stiffness and the number of swollen, tender joints in patients with RA. Fish oil supplementation may be beneficial for those with RA since it would be difficult to get to this level just from eating fish.

Grass-Fed and Pasture-Raised Animal Products

Many studies have shown that consuming meat from grass-fed animals provides far greater benefits than eating meat from an animal raised in a confined feeding operation with little or no outdoor access. Grass-fed animals are outside and exposed to sunlight, which increases their omega-3s and which has been shown to lead to a higher omega-3 content in the consumer's body.

Grass-fed beef also contains vitamins A, B_6, B_{12}, D, and E, and minerals such as zinc, iron, and selenium, and is an important source of essential amino acids, the building blocks of protein. Grass-fed beef has three times the amount of vitamin E than grain-fed beef!

For those with RA who can tolerate eggs, pasture-raised eggs come from chickens fully raised on the pasture and not confined indoors. The hen's diet influences the omega-3, vitamin, and mineral content of the egg. Studies have shown that eggs from pasture-raised hens compared to those housed in confinement had five times more vitamin A and 10 times more vitamin D.

Fish

I recommend consuming wild-caught fish because they come from their natural environment. Farm-raised fish are raised in pens, often with an unnatural diet. The data are not completely clear on whether wild-caught fish are higher in omega-3 fats than farmed fish, but there are other nutritional benefits: Wild-caught salmon has more vitamin D than farmed salmon (500 to 1,000 IU [international units] per 3.5 ounces versus 100 to 250 IU in 3.5 ounces of farmed salmon).

Nuts and Seeds

Plant sources of omega-3 fats include chia seeds, flaxseed, and walnuts. These contain the omega-3 fatty acid called alpha-linolenic acid (ALA), which also has anti-inflammatory effects. The compounds in flaxseed have been shown to inhibit atherosclerosis and reduce cholesterol levels. A healthy diet should have an approximate 1:4 ratio of omega-3 fats to omega-6 fats. Most omega-6 fats are more inflammatory than omega-3 fats and can be found in vegetable oils such as soybean and safflower, and processed foods.

Oils

Healthy oils include extra-virgin olive oil and virgin coconut oil. They contain a high amount of anti-inflammatory phenols. Inflammatory substances are produced in almost every tissue of the body, and phenols have the potential to block these to help keep inflammation under control.

VEGETABLES AND FRUITS

Vegetables and fruits provide fiber, are lower in calories, and contain powerful anti-inflammatory components (polyphenols) that help prevent chronic diseases.

The American Heart Association recommends 7 to 10 servings of fruits and vegetables per day. A serving size is 1 cup of a raw vegetable or ½ cup cooked. Aim for more servings of vegetables than fruit each day (5 servings of vegetables and 2 servings of fruits). This ensures you get great nutrition with a little less sugar from the fruit.

For most, berries (blackberries, blueberries, raspberries, strawberries) are great options because of their lower sugar content and anti-inflammatory benefits. Some people do not tolerate fruits well—they can be hard to digest with a compromised gut. If this is the case for you, try cooking the fruits to make them more easily digestible. For instance, make applesauce instead of eating raw apples.

Cruciferous vegetables are especially important as part of an anti-inflammatory diet. They include:

- Broccoli
- Brussel sprouts
- Cabbage
- Cauliflower
- Kale

They contain compounds called isothiocyanates, which inhibit NF-κB, a molecule that plays a central role in inflammation.

HERBS AND SPICES

Herbs and spices have incredible health benefits. They inhibit the pro-inflammatory pathways in the body, decreasing inflammation. The Quick Start Guide (page 5) lists five of my favorite herbs and spices and their benefits. You will find these used throughout the recipes in this book.

Add herbs and spices to your diet wherever you can. Herbal teas are wonderful to sip on throughout the day. Green tea contains polyphenols that help decrease inflammation in the body, and it also has antioxidant properties that prevent oxidative stress—preventing disease and damage to our cells.

Foods that Worsen Inflammation

Even though some individuals consume plenty of fruits and vegetables in their diets, which play a role in bringing down inflammation, they can still consume many foods that fuel the inflammatory cascade. I was one of them. Removing these inflammatory foods plays a pivotal role in health transformation:

pain diminishes, digestion improves, and energy increases. Many even report feeling happier! Here, we cover what those foods are and why they should be avoided.

SUGAR

The Obesity Society reports that adult consumption of added sugar in the United States has increased by more than 30 percent over three decades. Refined sugar lacks vitamins and minerals and has no nutritional value—and it can actually deplete us of nutrients when we digest it. For instance, chromium, an important mineral that plays a role in carbohydrate, fat, and protein metabolism, is needed to break down sugar, but unfortunately it can be depleted when we consume sugar.

White sugar leads to inflammation and changes our body chemistry. As little as two teaspoons of sugar can cause the nutrients to change and throw the blood chemistry out of balance. Imagine this happening day after day, year after year. The body becomes exhausted trying to get back into balance! In the case of a degenerative disease such as RA, the body is already having a hard time getting back in balance. Add sugar to the equation and we really have a problem.

We should be mindful of all forms of sugar in the diet, but one of the worst is high-fructose corn syrup. Beverages sweetened with high-fructose corn syrup have been shown to increase the risk of RA in women, independent of other dietary and lifestyle factors. Be mindful of other names for sugar added to foods:

- Brown sugar
- Corn sweetener
- Corn syrup
- Raw sugar
- Sugar molecules ending in *-ose* (dextrose, fructose, glucose, lactose, maltose, sucrose)
- Syrup

The good news is that chapter 10 (page 147) provides dessert recipes that offer nutritional value and satisfy your sweet tooth in a healthy way. Raw honey, an acceptable sweetener, is used. This is natural, unprocessed honey, which is a source of antioxidants, vitamins, and minerals and acts as an antimicrobial. Other acceptable sweeteners that should be consumed in moderation are stevia, coconut sugar, and 100% pure maple syrup.

FOOD SENSITIVITIES

As noted previously, there are also food sensitivities to consider when trying to keep inflammation in check.

Wheat Products
This group includes all white flour products, which should be avoided if you have an autoimmune disease such as RA. Many people with autoimmune diseases also have celiac disease or a nonceliac gluten sensitivity, where the body's immune system mistakes wheat protein as a foreigner. It mounts an antibody response that can cross-react with healthy tissue, damaging it systemically: joints, gut, liver, thyroid, heart, pancreas, bone, nervous system, and reproductive organs.

Dairy, Corn, and Other Grains
Following a gluten-free diet can offer sensitivity relief for many. However, not all people respond well to a gluten-free diet alone. Those who suffer from autoimmune conditions need to avoid much more than gluten, as proteins in other foods can cross-react with wheat proteins and cause your immune system to mount an attack against them. Research has shown that the proteins from corn, millet, milk, oats, and rice have a strong association with the antibodies produced against gliadin, one of the wheat proteins.

Many people with autoimmune conditions tolerate a few gluten-free grains: buckwheat, quinoa, and wild rice. You will find these in some recipes here. However, to prevent the body from reacting to their proteins, these grains should be consumed in small amounts and not every day.

As for flours, many people tolerate arrowroot, tapioca, nut flours (almond, hazelnut), and coconut flour, but again, this can vary based on an individual's sensitivities.

Coffee
Coffee is tolerable for some people with autoimmune conditions. Research has shown instant coffee may be traced with gluten and reacts more in individuals than pure coffee. As long as you do not have a coffee allergy, it may be fine to consume in small amounts, being mindful of what you put in it.

An Anti-Inflammatory Diet at a Glance

Food is medicine. It has powerful components that can help reduce the inflammatory process in our bodies. Here are handy lists of foods to enjoy and those to avoid on an anti-inflammatory diet.

Foods to Enjoy

FATS

- Avocado
- Beef, grass-fed
- Butter
- Coconut butter
- Coconut milk
- Coconut oil, virgin
- Eggs, pasture-raised, as tolerated
- Fish, wild-caught
- Ghee
- Guacamole
- Hummus
- Nuts (pecans, almonds, walnuts), as tolerated
- Nut butter (almond)
- Olive oil, extra-virgin
- Seeds (chia, flax, pumpkin, sunflower), as tolerated
- Seed butter (sunflower)

VEGETABLES

- All but the nightshades
- Cooked vegetables, which are more easily digested
- Non-starchy vegetables: asparagus, bok choy, broccoli, cabbage (green and purple), cauliflower, celery, collard greens, cucumbers, green beans, kale, radishes, spinach, sugar snap peas, zucchini
- Root vegetables: beets, carrots, parsnips, rutabaga, sweet potatoes, turnips

FRUITS

- Berries (blackberries, blueberries, rasp-berries, strawberries)
- Cooked fruits, as in homemade apple-sauce, may work well for some
- Other fruits as tolerated (you may notice you feel better when you avoid bananas, grapes, or other fruits that cause symptoms)

HERBS

- All are okay except those that contain peppers (cayenne pepper, paprika, red pepper flakes). These can aggravate some with RA.

SWEETENERS (IN MODERATION)

- Coconut sugar
- Honey, raw, if tolerated
- Maple syrup, 100% pure
- Stevia, which has no carcinogenic effect and a therapeutic effect against inflam-mation and diseases, including diabetes, cancer, and hypertension.

GRAINS (AS TOLERATED)

- Buckwheat (and cream of buckwheat, a great alternative to oatmeal)
- Quinoa
- Wild rice

LEGUMES (AS TOLERATED)

- Lentils
- Pinto beans

Foods to Avoid

DAIRY AND EGGS

- Dairy products, except butter and ghee
- Eggs (for some)

NOTE Some people with RA tolerate eggs, but they can be a problem for others. The immune system can cross-react with the protein found in eggs, causing a heightened immune response. Eggs provide a lot of great nutrition, but you may need to avoid them, at least for a period of time. I suggest first removing the main triggers: sugar, pasteurized dairy products, and the grains mentioned here. If you still have symptoms, avoid eggs for several weeks and see how you feel. The recipes in this book give you some egg-free ideas.

FATS

- Trans fats
- Vegetable oils

VEGETABLES

- Nightshade plants, including eggplant, okra, all peppers, white potatoes, sorrel, tomatillos, tomatoes

FRUITS

- Nightshade plants, including Goji berries, gooseberries

SPICES

- Cayenne pepper
- Paprika

NUTS

- Tree nuts (for some)

SWEETENERS

- White sugar

GRAINS

- Corn
- Flour, wheat and white
- Other grains not well tolerated, such as millet, oats, white and brown rice

LEGUMES

- Peanuts and other legumes, if not well tolerated

PROCESSED FOODS

- Processed meats
- Processed packaged foods

OTHER

- Coffee (for some)

Eggs

Eggs provide great nutrition, but those with an autoimmune condition may need to avoid them, at least for a period of time. The immune system could be cross-reacting with the protein found in eggs, causing a heightened immune response.

Peanuts and Other Legumes

Peanuts are in the legume family and, for many people with autoimmune conditions, should be avoided. Beans and lentils are also legumes and often not well tolerated in those with RA. Some people do fine with pinto beans and lentils but not black beans or soybeans.

Tree Nuts

Some people with RA have a sensitivity to tree nuts, which include almonds, Brazil nuts, cashews, pecans, and walnuts. Some people test fine for almonds and pecans but are sensitive to cashews and walnuts.

Trans Fats

We've already learned that trans fats are a type of manmade fat, altered to increase shelf life—and its nutrition labeling can be deceiving. The FDA does not require trans fat to be labeled if it is less than 0.5 grams per serving. So you could consume 0.4 grams of trans fat in one serving of crackers. This can add up if you eat more than one serving. Always look at the

Five Tips for Easier Home Cooking

Being in a state of chronic pain and fatigue can make home cooking challenging, but there are ways to make this easier.

BUY PRE-CUT VEGETABLES AND FRUITS to lessen the work done with your hands.

INVEST IN KITCHEN EQUIPMENT (it doesn't have to be expensive) that will save time and require less use of your hands: electric can opener, food processor, good set of knives, mandoline slicer.

PREPARE FOOD AHEAD OF TIME to save time in the kitchen (make a batch of sweet potatoes for the week or a pot of soup).

FLAG YOUR FAVORITE RECIPES so you can come back to them again easily.

PLAN YOUR MEALS, make a list, and stick to it. This will prevent several grocery shopping trips saving you time, energy, and money.

ingredient list for "partially hydrogenated oil," which means trans fat is in the product.

Vegetable Oils

Many vegetable oils are high in inflammatory omega-6 fats, leading to an increase in inflammation. These include oils made from corn, cottonseed, safflower and sunflower seeds, and soybeans. Vegetable oils are very fragile and, when processed and heated to high temperatures, become rancid quickly.

Processed Meats

These foods include breakfast sausages, canned meats, deli meats, and hot dogs. Processed meats have been shown to increase inflammation compared to unprocessed meats.

Animals raised in confined feeding operations and not grazing on pasture eat diets full of corn, soy, and grains. This reduces the healthy omega-3 fats in the meat and increases the pro-inflammatory omega-6 fats, which is what we then consume. The animals are also frequently given antibiotics and hormones, which we also consume when eating their meat.

To make matters worse, the corn and soy they're fed are often genetically modified (GM), meaning the plants' DNA has been modified through genetic engineering. Pigs fed a GM diet have been shown to have severe stomach inflammation compared to those fed a non-GMO diet. Imagine what eating their meat is doing to our insides.

Processed meats also typically contain preservatives such as nitrites and nitrates, which may form carcinogenic compounds when heated. While the evidence is inconsistent, it's better to consume meat without these additives. If you buy bacon, for example, buy the nitrate- and nitrite-free version.

Processed and Packaged Foods

These "dead foods" lack nutritional value because of the high amount of processing involved; they offer no anti-inflammatory benefit. They also contain harmful additives such as sugar, food dyes, artificial colorings, and preservatives.

Nightshades

These whole foods are healthy choices for most people, but those with RA may have a sensitivity to the chemicals they contain called alkaloids. Nightshades include eggplant, peppers, tobacco, tomatoes, and white potatoes. About one-third of arthritis sufferers who remove all nightshades from their diets feel some symptom relief.

The RA Pantry

The recipes in this book are designed to be easy to make and delicious. In the spirit of saving time, keeping a well-stocked pantry of essential items will save you from frequent and lengthy shopping trips.

MUST-HAVE PANTRY ITEMS

- Almond butter
- Bottled, minced garlic
- Coconut aminos (soy sauce substitute)
- Coconut milk, canned, full-fat and lite
- Dijon mustard

- Grain-free flours: almond, arrowroot, coconut, tapioca
- Honey, raw
- Nuts and seeds (not peanuts)
- Oils, extra-virgin olive and virgin coconut
- Tolerable legumes and grains: lentils, wild rice, quinoa, buckwheat
- Vanilla extract, pure
- Vegetable broth, low-sodium
- Vinegars, apple cider and balsamic

MUST-HAVE HERBS AND SPICES

- Black pepper
- Cilantro, fresh
- Cinnamon, ground
- Cloves, ground and whole
- Cumin, ground
- Garlic, bottled minced, fresh cloves, and powdered
- Ginger, fresh and ground
- Nutmeg, ground
- Rosemary, fresh
- Salt, good-quality (Kosher salt, Celtic sea salt, pink Himalayan salt) due to its higher nutritional and mineral content and less processing than white table salt
- Turmeric, ground

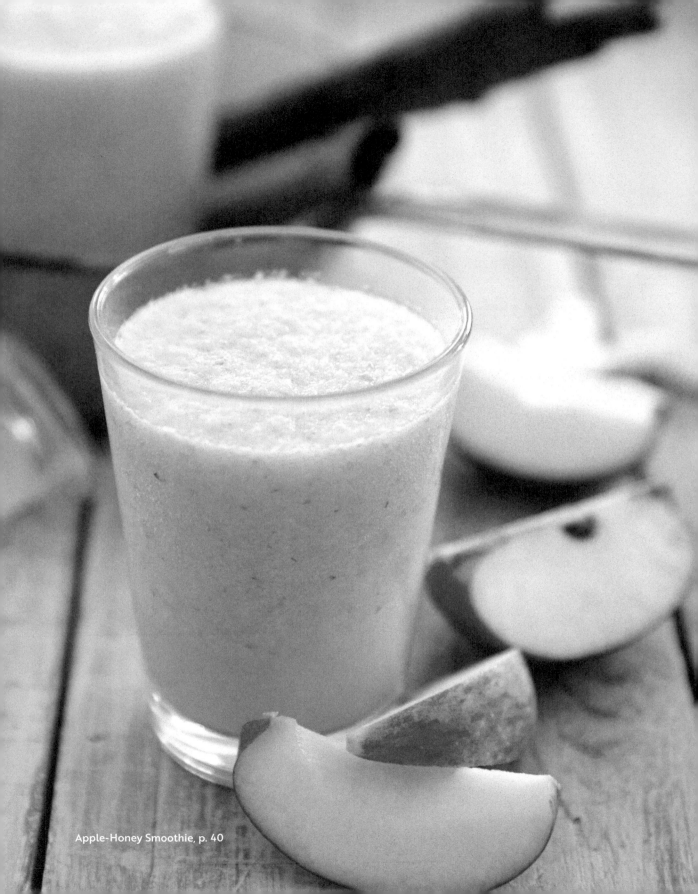

Apple-Honey Smoothie, p. 40

2

SMOOTHIES & BREAKFAST

CHAI SMOOTHIE

SERVES 2 **PREP** 5 minutes

The lovely mixed-spice scent of chai is often associated with hot tea, but this warm spice blend can also be delicious in a frothy cold drink. Brewed and cooled decaffeinated chai tea can be used here instead of the almond milk to create a more authentic taste. If you use the tea in this smoothie, omit the spices or reduce the amounts so the flavor is not overpowering.

Vegan

1 cup unsweetened almond milk

1 cup pure pumpkin purée

1 tablespoon pure maple syrup

1 teaspoon grated fresh peeled ginger

¼ teaspoon ground cinnamon

⅛ teaspoon ground nutmeg

Pinch ground cloves

Pinch ground cardamom

4 ice cubes

1. In a blender, combine the almond milk, pumpkin, maple syrup, ginger, cinnamon, nutmeg, cloves, and cardamom. Blend until smooth.

2. Add the ice and blend until thick.

INGREDIENT TIP Canned pumpkin products are fine, but try roasting a pumpkin yourself for lovely flavor and control over additives. Cool any excess pumpkin and freeze it for up to 2 months for future use.

PER SERVING Calories: 88; Total fat: 2g; Saturated fat: 0g; Carbohydrates: 18g; Fiber: 4g; Protein: 2g

"CHOCOLATE"-AVOCADO SMOOTHIE

SERVES 2 **PREP** 5 minutes

Although chocolate is not actually used to flavor this thick beverage, carob makes a lovely substitute—without the caffeine and theobromine that can exacerbate rheumatoid arthritis. Carob has more fiber and less fat than chocolate and a whopping three times the amount of calcium. Carob does not taste exactly like chocolate, but you will not be disappointed with the flavor and chocolate-y color of this smoothie.

Vegetarian

1 cup unsweetened almond milk

1 cup shredded kale

½ avocado

½ banana

2 tablespoons carob powder

1 tablespoon coconut oil

1 tablespoon raw honey

1 teaspoon pure vanilla extract

4 ice cubes

1. In a blender, combine the almond milk, kale, avocado, banana, carob powder, coconut oil, honey, and vanilla. Blend until smooth.

2. Add the ice and blend until thick.

INGREDIENT TIP Carob can be found in the organic or health section of the supermarket. This ingredient can be used in a 1:1 ratio wherever you see chocolate in a recipe.

PER SERVING Calories: 295; Total fat: 19g; Saturated fat: 10g; Carbohydrates: 27g; Fiber: 5g; Protein: 3g

MINTY GREEN SMOOTHIE

SERVES 2 **PREP** 5 minutes

Avocado is a fabulous smoothie ingredient because it creates a velvety milkshake-like texture and adds many nutritional benefits such as healthy fats, potassium, and fiber. The monounsaturated fat in avocados can improve the absorption of the carotenoids found in the spinach. This absorption rate increases four to six times the usual rate, and avocados can also improve the conversion of carotenoids to disease-fighting vitamin A.

Vegetarian

1 cup canned lite coconut milk

1 cup fresh spinach

1 banana, cut into chunks

½ avocado

½ English cucumber, cut into chunks

2 tablespoons chopped fresh mint

1 tablespoon freshly squeezed lemon juice

1 tablespoon raw honey

3 ice cubes

1. In a blender, combine the coconut milk, spinach, banana, avocado, cucumber, mint, lemon juice, and honey. Blend until smooth.

2. Add the ice and blend until thick.

COOKING TIP Mint comes in huge bunches that contain too much for just this smoothie. Chop the remaining mint finely, scoop it into an ice cube tray, and add water to fill the compartments. Freeze the mint cubes and just pop them into the smoothie instead of plain ice cubes. Two cubes would equal the amount of fresh mint called for in this recipe.

PER SERVING Calories: 482; Total fat: 40g; Saturated fat: 28g; Carbohydrates: 37g; Fiber: 9g; Protein: 6g

CREAMY PISTACHIO SMOOTHIE

SERVES 2 **PREP** 5 minutes

If you are a fan of pistachio ice cream, this is the smoothie for you. If you want a crunchy texture similar to the ice cream, add the pistachios at the end instead and pulse to chop rather than purée. Remember to remove the skins on the bananas before freezing them. Otherwise, you'll have to cut off the frozen black skins, which is a fiddly task.

Vegan

1 cup unsweetened almond milk

1 cup shredded kale

2 frozen bananas

½ cup shelled pistachios

2 tablespoons pure maple syrup

1 teaspoon pure vanilla extract

In a blender, combine the milk, kale, bananas, pistachios, maple syrup, and vanilla. Blend until smooth and thick.

INGREDIENT TIP Pistachios can be found in a pretty natural greenish color or an incredibly vibrant red, which is obviously dyed. Always reach for the natural pistachios to avoid unhealthy preservatives and to keep your smoothie green.

PER SERVING Calories: 275; Total fat: 4g; Saturated fat: 1g; Carbohydrates: 48g; Fiber: 5g; Protein: 6g

TROPICAL RED SMOOTHIE

SERVES 2 **PREP** 5 minutes

For a truly tropical experience, toss in a cup of diced mango or papaya along with the other fruit. The extra fruit will not add too many more calories to the smoothie (1 cup of mango adds 53 calories per serving and papaya adds 27 calories per serving), however, it will increase the sugar load of the smoothie. If your goal is weight loss, you will want to keep the sugar intake down and add in more protein and greens for balance—such as a scoop of good-quality protein powder and a handful of spinach leaves. You will still be delighted with the sunrise hue of this energy-packed breakfast.

Vegan

1 cup coconut water

½ cup unsweetened pineapple juice

1 banana

½ cup fresh raspberries

½ cup unsweetened shredded coconut

3 ice cubes

1. In a blender, combine the coconut water, pineapple juice, banana, raspberries, and coconut. Blend until smooth.

2. Add the ice and blend until thick.

SUBSTITUTION TIP Coconut water can be found in most grocery stores in the health food section, but if you find yourself without this ingredient, an equal amount of unsweetened apple juice or water can be used in place of the coconut water.

PER SERVING Calories: 209; Total fat: 10g; Saturated fat: 8g; Carbohydrates: 31g; Fiber: 7g; Protein: 3g

SWEET POTATO PIE SMOOTHIE

SERVES 2 **PREP** 5 minutes

Sweet potato pie, a Southern staple, is similar to pumpkin pie with a hint of orange and salt. The ingredients in this bright smoothie taste close to the pastry version, but without the added fat and sugar. For an extra-rich flavor, toast the pumpkin seeds in a low-heat oven until crispy and fragrant before adding them to the blender. If weight loss is your goal, you can reduce the banana and orange juice quantities in half and add in a little more unsweetened almond milk. While these are foods that contain natural sugars, we still want to be mindful of the effect they can have on weight loss.

Vegan

½ cup unsweetened almond milk

½ cup freshly squeezed orange juice

1 cup cooked sweet potato

1 banana

2 tablespoons pumpkin seeds

1 tablespoon pure maple syrup

½ teaspoon pure vanilla extract

½ teaspoon ground cinnamon

3 ice cubes

1. In a blender, combine the almond milk, orange juice, sweet potato, banana, pumpkin seeds, maple syrup, vanilla, and cinnamon. Blend until smooth.

2. Add the ice and blend until thick.

COOKING TIP Sweet potatoes are packed with nutrients and can be used in a multitude of culinary applications, especially if you have cooked sweet potatoes on hand. Baked sweet potatoes can be kept in their skins in the refrigerator for up to 5 days, so make some ahead for this recipe and others.

PER SERVING Calories: 235; Total fat: 4g; Saturated fat: 1g; Carbohydrates: 43g; Fiber: 6g; Protein: 5g

APPLE-HONEY SMOOTHIE

SERVES 2 **PREP** 5 minutes

Apple wedges topped with a dollop of nut butter are an outstanding healthy snack, so it makes sense to combine those ingredients in a tempting smoothie. Honey and banana add a delightful sweetness, and cinnamon creates a warm, fragrant finish. Leaving the skin on the apple is the best way to optimize the soluble fiber—pectin—in this popular fruit. Just make sure to scrub the apples well, even if they are organic. If weight loss is your goal, you can reduce the amount of banana by half to cut back on some of the sugar load.

Vegetarian

1 cup canned lite coconut milk

1 apple, cored and cut into chunks

1 banana

¼ cup almond butter

1 tablespoon raw honey

½ teaspoon ground cinnamon

4 ice cubes

1. In a blender, combine the coconut milk, apple, banana, almond butter, honey, and cinnamon. Blend until smooth.

2. Add the ice and blend until thick.

VARIATION TIP Ripe pears are a perfect choice if you want to try fruit other than apples in this beverage. Using pears adds only 4 calories as well as a little extra fiber and protein.

PER SERVING Calories: 434; Total fat: 30g; Saturated fat: 26g; Carbohydrates: 46g; Fiber: 8g; Protein: 4g

FRUIT-AND-SEED BREAKFAST BARS

SERVES 6 **PREP** 15 minutes **COOK** 30 minutes

The variety of seeds and dried fruit found in these pretty, golden bars makes them extremely filling and loaded with satisfying texture. Slivered and chopped nuts, such as cashews or almonds, could also be delectable if you want to replace one type of seed. Add the chopped nuts with the almond butter so they stay in larger chunks for an appealing look and crunchy bite.

Make Ahead

Vegan

½ cup pitted dates

¾ cup toasted sunflower seeds

¾ cup toasted pumpkin seeds

¾ cup white sesame seeds

½ cup dried blueberries

½ cup dried cherries

¼ cup flaxseed

½ cup almond butter

1. Preheat the oven to 325°F.

2. Line an 8-by-8-inch baking dish with parchment paper.

3. In a food processor, pulse the dates until chopped into a paste.

4. Add the sunflower seeds, pumpkin seeds, sesame seeds, blueberries, cherries, and flaxseed, and pulse to combine. Scoop the mixture into a medium bowl.

5. Stir in the almond butter. Transfer the mixture to the prepared dish and press it down firmly.

6. Bake for about 30 minutes, or until firm and golden brown.

7. Cool for about 1 hour, until it is at room temperature. Remove from the baking dish and cut into 12 squares.

8. Refrigerate in a sealed container for up to 1 week.

SUBSTITUTION TIP Any dried fruit can be used in place of the blueberries or cherries as long as the substitutions are sugar-free and preservative-free. Try apple, mango, currants, or papaya for a different taste.

PER SERVING (2 bars) Calories: 312; Total fat: 22g; Saturated fat: 4g; Carbohydrates: 24g, Fiber: 6g; Protein: 10g

CHIA-COCONUT PORRIDGE

SERVES 4 **PREP** 5 minutes plus 30 minutes soaking

Porridge is often thought to be a hot oatmeal or grain mixture, but the definition can stretch to include this creamy cold breakfast dish. You might be reminded of Cream of Wheat or tapioca when you experience the texture of soaked chia, thick with tiny bubbles or balls. Chia seeds have more protein and healthy fats than grain cereals and 10 times the fiber. Keep this nutritious porridge in the refrigerator for a handy snack and a speedy breakfast option.

Make Ahead

Vegetarian

¾ cup water

¾ cup unsweetened almond milk

1 teaspoon pure vanilla extract

¼ cup chia seeds

¼ cup unsweetened shredded coconut

2 tablespoons raw honey

½ cup sliced fresh strawberries

1. In a medium bowl, whisk the water, almond milk, and vanilla until well blended.

2. Stir in the chia seeds, cover the bowl, and refrigerate it for a minimum of 30 minutes and up to overnight.

3. Stir the coconut and honey into the chilled porridge. Spoon the porridge into four bowls.

4. Serve topped with the strawberries.

INGREDIENT TIP Chia seeds come in black and white, or a mix of the two, depending on the brand. Nutritionally they are similar, with a little less protein and more fiber in the black, but the white chia seeds are much more visually appealing in this pretty porridge.

PER SERVING Calories: 124; Total fat: 7g; Saturated fat: 4g; Carbohydrates: 15g; Fiber: 4g; Protein: 2g

GOLDEN COCONUT PANCAKES

SERVES 4 **PREP** 10 minutes **COOK** 10 minutes

Stacks of steaming fluffy pancakes with maple syrup or sweet berries are the epitome of a picture-perfect weekend breakfast. These are so simple you can enjoy them during the week as well. If you have leftover pancakes or want to make a double batch, wrap and refrigerate the extras, after they have cooled, for up to five days. Pop the pancakes in the toaster to reheat and enjoy.

Vegan

½ cup almond flour

¼ cup coconut flour

1 teaspoon baking soda

3 eggs, beaten

2 bananas, mashed

1 teaspoon pure vanilla extract

1 tablespoon coconut oil

Pure maple syrup, for serving (optional)

Fresh fruit, for serving (optional)

1. In a medium bowl, stir together the almond flour, coconut flour, and baking soda until well mixed.

2. Make a well in the center and add the eggs, bananas, and vanilla. Beat together until well blended.

3. Place a large skillet over medium-high heat and add the coconut oil.

4. For each pancake, pour ¼ cup of batter into the skillet, four per batch. Cook for about 3 minutes, or until the bottom is golden and the bubbles on the surface burst. Flip and cook for about 2 minutes more until golden and cooked through. Transfer to a plate and repeat with any remaining batter.

5. Serve with a drizzle of maple syrup or top with fresh fruit (if using).

INGREDIENT TIP Coconut flour is a different ingredient to bake with, especially if you have not used it before. Do not cut back on the eggs and other liquid in this recipe, because coconut flour is ultra absorbent and requires a great deal of moisture.

PER SERVING (2 pancakes) Calories: 218; Total fat: 15g; Saturated fat: 6g; Carbohydrates: 17g; Fiber: 4g; Protein: 8g

MINI BROCCOLI FRITTATAS

SERVES 4 **PREP** 10 minutes **COOK** 20 minutes

Chopped broccoli and spinach produce a striking green-flecked egg dish that can be eaten with a knife and fork while piping hot, or carried cold as you run out the door in the morning. Broccoli is extremely high in vitamins K and C as well as fiber and phosphorus. This recipe does not use an entire head of broccoli, so just cut off the amount needed and place the rest in the refrigerator without washing or preparing it, which helps preserve its levels of vitamin C.

Make Ahead

Vegetarian

Olive oil, for greasing the muffin cups

8 eggs

¼ cup unsweetened almond milk

½ teaspoon chopped fresh basil

½ cup chopped broccoli

½ cup shredded fresh spinach

1 scallion, white and green parts, chopped

Pinch sea salt

Pinch freshly ground black pepper

1. Preheat the oven to 350°F.

2. Lightly oil a 6-cup muffin tin and set it aside.

3. In a medium bowl, whisk the eggs, almond milk, and basil until frothy.

4. Stir in the broccoli, spinach, and scallion. Spoon the egg mixture into the muffin cups.

5. Bake for about 20 minutes, or until the frittatas are puffed, golden, and cooked through.

6. Season with sea salt and pepper and serve.

COOKING TIP This entire recipe can be put together, poured into the muffin cups, and refrigerated without baking. In the morning, just pop the tray right from the refrigerator into a preheated oven to bake and enjoy.

PER SERVING Calories: 132; Total fat: 9g; Saturated fat: 3g; Carbohydrates: 2g; Fiber: 1g; Protein: 12g

EGG CASSEROLE WITH SWEET POTATO AND KALE

SERVES 4 **PREP** 15 minutes **COOK** 30 minutes

Lazy weekend mornings call for a dish that can be thrown together and baked up like a fine-dining brunch menu item. This colorful creation bursts with an assortment of vegetables, fragrant spices, and fresh herbs. Serve a generous portion with a fresh fruit salad and a steaming cup of herbal tea or freshly squeezed orange juice. Leftovers make a filling lunch the next day, either hot or cold.

Make Ahead

Vegetarian

Olive oil, for greasing the baking dish

1 cup diced cooked sweet potato

1 cup chopped blanched cauliflower

1 cup shredded kale

1 scallion, white and green parts, chopped

1 teaspoon chopped fresh basil

8 eggs

¼ cup unsweetened almond milk

1 teaspoon ground cumin

1 teaspoon ground coriander

Pinch sea salt

Pinch freshly ground black pepper

1. Preheat the oven to 375°F.

2. Lightly grease a 9-by-13-inch baking dish with olive oil.

3. Evenly spread the sweet potato, cauliflower, kale, scallion, and basil in the prepared dish.

4. In a medium bowl, whisk the eggs, almond milk, cumin, coriander, sea salt, and pepper. Pour the egg mixture into the baking dish, lightly tapping the dish on the counter to distribute the eggs among the vegetables.

5. Bake for about 30 minutes, or until the eggs are set and the top is lightly golden.

VARIATION TIP Casseroles are incredibly forgiving, so you can swap out, or in, almost any ingredient to create an interesting dish. For example, the sweet potato can be pumpkin or squash and the kale could be changed to spinach. Chopped cooked chicken would also be a tasty addition.

PER SERVING Calories: 206; Total fat: 10g; Saturated fat: 3g; Carbohydrates: 15g; Fiber: 3g; Protein: 15g

SWEET POTATO-GROUND TURKEY HASH

SERVES 4 **PREP** 10 minutes **COOK** 26 minutes

Hash is traditionally made with corned beef, or but as it is cured in salt it is inappropriate for most healthy diets. The ground turkey used here, because it is mild and juicy, combines beautifully with sweet potato and warm spices. Look for extra-lean meat, about 93 percent lean for the best results.

1½ pounds extra-lean ground turkey

1 sweet onion, chopped, or about 1 cup precut packaged onion

2 teaspoons bottled minced garlic

1 teaspoon ground ginger

2 pounds sweet potatoes, peeled, cooked, and diced

Pinch sea salt

Pinch freshly ground black pepper

Pinch ground cloves

1 cup chopped kale

1. In a large skillet over medium-high heat, sauté the turkey for about 10 minutes, or until it is cooked through.

2. Add the onion, garlic, and ginger. Sauté for 3 minutes.

3. Add the sweet potatoes, sea salt, pepper, and cloves. Reduce the heat to medium. Sauté for about 10 minutes, stirring until the sweet potato is heated through.

4. Stir in the kale. Cook for about 3 minutes, stirring until it has wilted.

5. Divide the hash among four bowls and serve.

SUBSTITUTION TIP Homemade sausage or sausage with no preservatives is a nice alternative to turkey. Read the labels carefully to source the best ingredients.

PER SERVING Calories: 467; Total fat: 14g; Saturated fat: 4g; Carbohydrates: 50g; Fiber: 8g; Protein: 34g

GROUND BEEF BREAKFAST SKILLET

SERVES 4 **PREP** 20 minutes **COOK** 20 minutes

Once you get past the idea that you are having ground beef for breakfast, this satisfying dish might become your new favorite way to start the day. The combination of protein and a plethora of healthy vegetable carbs keep you feeling full until lunch. Any vegetable would be delicious, so feel free to experiment with your favorites.

1 tablespoon olive oil

1 pound lean ground beef

2 teaspoons bottled minced garlic

2 cups chopped cauliflower

1 cup diced carrots

1 zucchini, diced

2 scallions, white and green parts, chopped

Sea salt

Freshly ground black pepper

2 tablespoons chopped fresh parsley

1. Place a large skillet over medium-high heat and add the olive oil.

2. Add the ground beef and garlic. Sauté for about 8 minutes, or until cooked through.

3. Stir in the cauliflower, carrots, and zucchini. Sauté for about 10 minutes, or until tender.

4. Stir in the scallions and sauté for 1 minute more.

5. Season the mixture with sea salt and pepper. Serve topped with the parsley.

SUBSTITUTION TIP The cauliflower can be replaced with cabbage if you prefer. Try preshredded cabbage found in packages in the salad section of the supermarket.

PER SERVING Calories: 214; Total fat: 9g; Saturated fat: 3g; Carbohydrates: 7g; Fiber: 2g; Protein: 26g

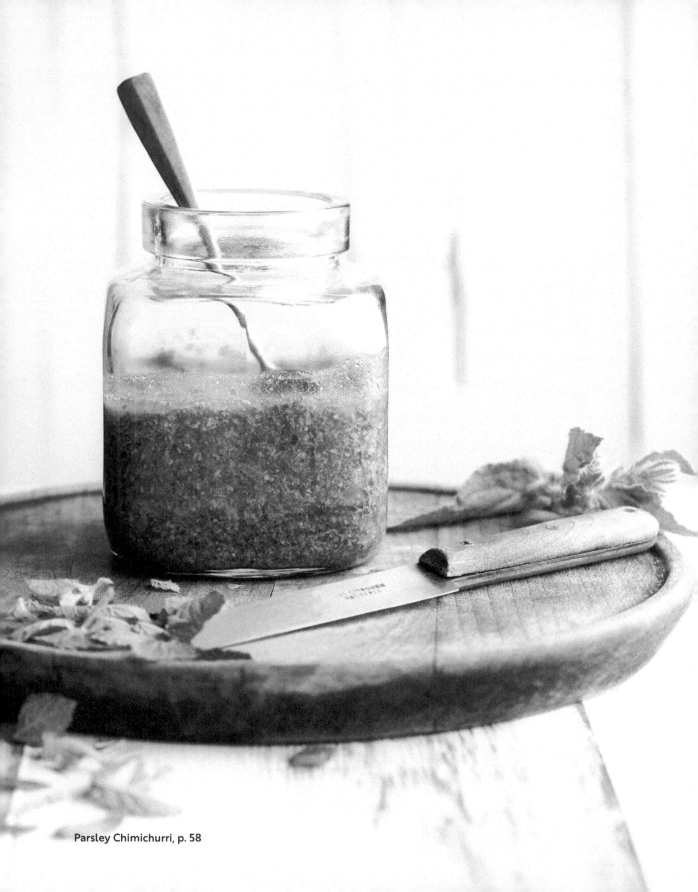

Parsley Chimichurri, p. 58

3

CONDIMENTS, DRESSINGS & SAUCES

MILD CURRY POWDER

MAKES ¼ cup   **PREP** 5 minutes

Commercially prepared curry powders usually contain many of the nightshade spices not recommended for rheumatoid arthritis, such as cayenne pepper and paprika. This flavorful blend is composed of acceptable spices, and the resulting curry powder is delicious and versatile. So continue to enjoy all those curry-based dishes you love.

Make Ahead
Vegan

1 tablespoon
ground turmeric

1 tablespoon ground cumin

2 teaspoons
ground coriander

1 teaspoon
ground cardamom

1 teaspoon ground cinnamon

1 teaspoon ground ginger

½ teaspoon
fenugreek powder

½ teaspoon ground cloves

1. In a small bowl, stir together the turmeric, cumin, coriander, cardamom, cinnamon, ginger, fenugreek, and cloves until well blended.

2. Store the curry powder in an airtight container for up to 1 month.

COOKING TIP For stronger flavor, purchase cumin and coriander seeds and grind your own spices in a coffee grinder or with a mortar and pestle. You can also lightly toast the seeds first to create a truly sublime spice blend.

PER SERVING (1 teaspoon) Calories: 6; Total fat: 0g; Saturated fat: 0g; Carbohydrates: 1g; Fiber: 0g; Protein: 0g

MEDITERRANEAN RUB

MAKES ¾ cup   **PREP** 5 minutes

Spice and herb rubs are one of the simplest methods to create flavorful meats, poultry, and fish with very few added calories or fat. The coconut sugar here, which is only a very small amount considering the portion size, helps with caramelization. Coconut sugar can be found in the organic section of most supermarkets, or source it in bulk or from health food stores.

Make Ahead

Vegan

¼ cup packed coconut sugar

3 tablespoons dried oregano leaves

2 tablespoons dried thyme leaves

1 tablespoon dried tarragon

1 teaspoon dried marjoram

1 teaspoon dried dill

1 teaspoon dried basil

1. In a small bowl, stir together the coconut sugar, oregano, thyme, tarragon, marjoram, dill, and basil until well blended.

2. Store the seasoning in a sealed container for up to 1 month.

SUBSTITUTION TIP The dried herbs in this seasoning blend are not the only choices that work together. To maintain a Mediterranean taste in the mixture, keep the oregano because it is a very popular herb in that region's cuisines.

PER SERVING (1 teaspoon) Calories: 5; Total fat: 0g; Saturated fat: 0g; Carbohydrates: 1g; Fiber: 0g; Protein: 0g

SPICY TUNISIAN VINAIGRETTE

MAKES 1¼ cups   **PREP** 5 minutes

A tasty never-fail vinaigrette recipe is a culinary necessity, especially when you are trying to eat healthy or follow a specific diet. This dressing has a warm spice kick and a hint of citrus to perk up your taste buds. If you want to keep it longer than a couple weeks, use ⅛ teaspoon garlic powder instead of 1 teaspoon minced garlic. This vinaigrette can also be prepared in a blender if you do not want to whisk it.

Make Ahead
Vegan

¾ cup olive oil

¼ cup apple cider vinegar

1 tablespoon freshly squeezed lemon juice

¼ cup chopped fresh parsley

1 teaspoon bottled minced garlic

1 teaspoon ground cumin

¼ teaspoon ground coriander

Pinch sea salt

1. In a medium bowl, whisk the olive oil, cider vinegar, and lemon juice until emulsified.

2. Whisk in the parsley, garlic, cumin, and coriander.

3. Season with sea salt.

4. Refrigerate the vinaigrette in a sealed container for up to 2 weeks.

VARIATION TIP Apple cider vinegar is a slightly sweet, golden product that can be replaced with balsamic vinegar if you want a more robust vinaigrette. Try fig or maple balsamic vinegar for added flavor.

PER SERVING (2 tablespoons) Calories: 133; Total fat: 15g; Saturated fat: 2g; Carbohydrates: 0g; Fiber: 0g; Protein: 0g

CREAMY SESAME DRESSING

MAKES ¾ cup **PREP** 5 minutes

You might be wondering what you could use this rich sesame dressing for, but a better question might be what can't you top with this dressing? Vegetables, salad, grilled chicken, baked fish, and even a tasty breakfast casserole can all be enhanced with a little drizzle of toasty sesame flavor. If you enjoy sesame as an ingredient, make a quick and easy tahini paste in a blender with just sesame seeds and olive oil.

Make Ahead

Vegan

½ cup canned full-fat coconut milk

2 tablespoons tahini

2 tablespoons freshly squeezed lime juice

1 teaspoon bottled minced garlic

1 teaspoon minced fresh chives

Pinch sea salt

1. In a small bowl, whisk the coconut milk, tahini, lime juice, garlic, and chives until well blended. You can also prepare this in a blender.

2. Season with sea salt and transfer the dressing to a container with a lid. Refrigerate for up to 1 week.

COOKING TIP Fresh minced garlic is lovely, but if you use a great deal of this ingredient, it would be more efficient to purchase your garlic already minced. Just check the date on the jar, and do not let it sit too long in the refrigerator before finishing it off.

PER SERVING (1 tablespoon) Calories: 40; Total fat: 4g; Saturated fat: 2g; Carbohydrates: 2g; Fiber: 0g; Protein: 1g

MAPLE DRESSING

MAKES 1¼ cups   **PREP** 5 minutes

Maple syrup is a scrumptious ingredient made from the sap collected from sugar maple trees that grow in America's northeast and eastern Canada during a four- to six-week period around the end of March. Always refrigerate or freeze maple syrup to keep it fresh and delicious.

Make Ahead

Vegan

1 cup canned full-fat coconut milk

2 tablespoons pure maple syrup

1 tablespoon Dijon mustard

1 tablespoon apple cider vinegar

Sea salt

1. In a medium bowl, whisk the coconut milk, maple syrup, mustard, and cider vinegar until smoothly blended. Season with sea salt. You can also prepare this in a blender.

2. Refrigerate the dressing in a sealed container for up to 1 week.

INGREDIENT TIP Read the label on your maple syrup carefully to make sure the product is pure. Some maple syrups are cut with other ingredients, such as corn syrup or table syrup, to save money.

PER SERVING (2 tablespoons) Calories: 67; Total fat: 6g; Saturated fat: 5g; Carbohydrates: 4g; Fiber: 1g; Protein: 1g

AVOCADO-HERB SPREAD

MAKES 1 cup   **PREP** 10 minutes

Lemon juice does more than keep this creamy spread from turning an unsightly grayish color due to oxidization; it also adds a hefty nutritional punch and brings out the flavor of the other ingredients. Lemons are packed with antioxidants such as vitamin C and phyto-nutrients, which help fight cancer, detox the body, and boost the immune system. High doses of vitamin C have also been linked to protection against rheumatoid arthritis.

Make Ahead

Vegan

1 avocado, peeled and pitted

2 tablespoons freshly squeezed lemon juice

2 tablespoons chopped fresh parsley

1 teaspoon chopped fresh dill

½ teaspoon ground coriander

Sea salt

Freshly ground black pepper

1. In a blender, pulse the avocado until smoothly puréed.

2. Add the lemon juice, parsley, dill, and coriander. Pulse until well blended.

3. Season with sea salt and pepper.

4. Refrigerate the spread in a sealed container for up to 4 days.

COOKING TIP Ripe avocado is crucial for the correct texture here, but sometimes it is difficult to find fruit at the perfect stage of softness. To speed the ripening process, seal the avocado in a paper bag with a banana or apple for 2 to 3 days.

PER SERVING (2 tablespoons) Calories: 53; Total fat: 5g; Saturated fat: 1g; Carbohydrates: 2g; Fiber: 2g; Protein: 1g

PEACH BUTTER

MAKES 2 cups   **PREP** 10 minutes   **COOK** 3 hours, 30 minutes

Peaches are a fragrant fruit that come as freestone or clingstone varieties, either of which work beautifully for this recipe. If you want a set-it-and-forget-it method of making peach butter, use a slow cooker instead of cooking it on the stove top. Purée the peaches with the honey in a food processor, and pour the mixture into a cooker. Cook on low for 3 to 6 hours with the lid propped open a little so the peaches don't scorch.

Make Ahead

Vegetarian

8 peaches (about 3 pounds), peeled, pitted, and chopped, or about 6 cups frozen, sliced peaches

Water, for cooking

¼ cup raw honey

1. In a large saucepan over high heat, combine the peaches with enough water to cover the fruit by about 1 inch. Bring the liquid to a boil.

2. Reduce the heat to low and simmer for about 3 hours, stirring frequently until the mixture resembles a thick applesauce.

3. Stir in the honey. Simmer for about 30 minutes until the mixture starts to caramelize. Remove the peach butter from the heat and let it cool for 30 minutes.

4. Spoon the mixture into a container and cool completely before covering. Keep refrigerated for up to 2 weeks.

SUBSTITUTION TIP Peaches create a luscious, sweet spread when reduced to butter, but almost any fruit is also lovely. Try plums, cherries, apples, or pears as well as combinations of fruit until you hit upon your favorite flavor.

PER SERVING (2 tablespoons) Calories: 46; Total fat: 0g; Saturated fat: 0g; Carbohydrates: 11g; Fiber: 1g; Protein: 1g

SWEET CARROT SPREAD

MAKES 2 cups   **PREP** 10 minutes

The vibrant color of this spread will certainly add something special to your snacks or sandwiches made with gluten-free bread. The lovely, sweet flavor is spectacular combined with turkey or roast chicken and topped with shredded kale. Try dipping apple wedges or other fruit into this spread for a nutritious snack when you need an energy boost in the middle of a hectic day.

Make Ahead
Vegan

3 carrots, peeled and cut into chunks

½ cup almonds

2 tablespoons freshly squeezed lemon juice

1 tablespoon pure maple syrup

½ teaspoon ground cardamom

Sea salt

1. In a food processor, pulse the carrots until very finely chopped.

2. Add the almonds, lemon juice, maple syrup, and cardamom. Process until smooth.

3. Season the spread with sea salt and transfer to a lidded container. Refrigerate for up to 6 days.

COOKING TIP If you want a velvety smooth spread, use cooked carrots instead of raw. This reduces the storing time to 3 days so if you opt for cooked vegetables, make sure to use the spread quickly.

PER SERVING (2 tablespoons) Calories: 26; Total fat: 2g; Saturated fat: 0g; Carbohydrates: 3g; Fiber: 1g; Protein: 1g

PARSLEY CHIMICHURRI

MAKES 1 cup   **PREP** 5 minutes

This version of chimichurri is definitely classed as the green (verde) type. There is also a red (rojo) version featuring tomatoes, red pepper, and red pepper flakes. Chimichurri can be spooned over meats, fish, poultry, and vegetables, but it also makes a lovely marinade. Just whip up a batch, and pour it into a sealable plastic bag with whatever ingredient you are preparing for your meal. Place the bag in the refrigerator for one hour, and discard the marinade before broiling or grilling the protein.

Make Ahead

Vegan

1 cup coarsely chopped fresh parsley

½ cup fresh mint leaves

¼ cup olive oil

2 tablespoons freshly squeezed lemon juice

2 teaspoons bottled minced garlic

Pinch sea salt

1. In a blender or food processor, combine the parsley, mint, olive oil, lemon juice, garlic, and sea salt. Pulse until the herbs are very finely chopped and the ingredients are well mixed.

2. Refrigerate the mixture in a sealed container for up to 1 week.

VARIATION TIP Basil, oregano, mint, savory, and cilantro can all be used instead for this chimichurri if parsley is not your favorite herb. Mixtures of different herbs make a lovely sauce as well.

PER SERVING (2 tablespoons) Calories: 61; Total fat: 6g; Saturated fat: 1g; Carbohydrates: 1g; Fiber: 1g; Protein: 1g

TRADITIONAL GREMOLATA SAUCE

MAKES 1 cup   **PREP** 10 minutes

You will be delighted with the number of ways this flavorful sauce can be used to dress up your meals. Spoon it over meat, poultry, and fish for a main course, or add a little extra olive oil and create a fresh-tasting salad dressing. Gremolata can be tossed with vegetable noodles as you would pesto, and the sauce makes a flavorful marinade or rub before grilling or broiling chicken or pork. You just might want to make a double batch!

Make Ahead
Vegan

¾ cup finely chopped fresh parsley

Juice of 2 lemons (or 6 tablespoons)

Zest of 2 lemons (optional)

2 tablespoons olive oil

2 teaspoons bottled minced garlic

¼ teaspoon sea salt

1. In a small bowl, stir together the parsley, lemon juice, lemon zest (if using), olive oil, garlic, and sea salt until well blended.

2. Refrigerate in a sealed container for up to 4 days.

COOKING TIP There is something almost hypnotic about chopping a huge pile of fresh parsley by hand with a knife. If you don't have the time or your hands hurt today, use a blender or food processor to get the right texture.

PER SERVING (2 tablespoons) Calories: 33; Total fat: 4g; Saturated fat: 1g; Carbohydrates: 1g; Fiber: 0g; Protein: 0g

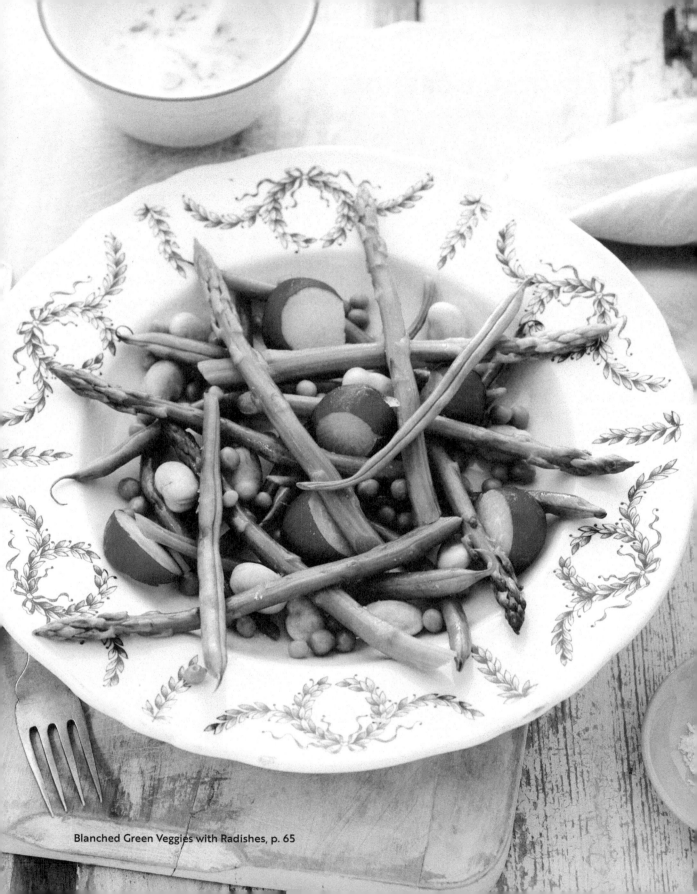

Blanched Green Veggies with Radishes, p. 65

4

VEGETABLES & SIDES

KALE-STUFFED MUSHROOMS

SERVES 4 **PREP** 15 minutes **COOK** 28 minutes

A perfect side for a grilled steak, or an inspired appetizer for an intimate get-together with family and friends. There is something utterly charming about mushroom caps, almost fairy-tale-like, especially when stuffed with dark green herbs and kale as well as pale artichoke hearts. To reduce the chopping, use a food processor for the ingredients prep (but pulse only a very few times or the vegetables will be too fine), stuff the mushrooms ahead of time, and bake them just before serving to save time and cleanup.

Vegan

16 large white button mushrooms, stemmed

2 teaspoons olive oil

½ cup finely chopped sweet onion

1 teaspoon bottled minced garlic

2 cups finely shredded kale

1 cup chopped water-packed canned artichoke hearts

1 teaspoon chopped fresh basil

1 teaspoon chopped fresh oregano

⅛ teaspoon sea salt

1. Preheat the oven to 375°F.

2. Arrange the mushroom caps, hollow-side up, on a baking sheet.

3. Place a large skillet over medium-high heat and add the olive oil.

4. Add the onion and garlic. Sauté for about 3 minutes, or until tender.

5. Stir in the kale, artichoke hearts, basil, oregano, and sea salt. Sauté for about 5 minutes, or until the kale is wilted.

6. With the back of a spoon, squeeze the liquid out of the filling into the skillet and evenly divide the mixture among the mushroom caps.

7. Bake for about 20 minutes, or until the mushrooms are tender. Serve warm.

INGREDIENT TIP Canned artichoke hearts are a convenient and delicious choice for people who love this vegetable but do not want to handle a raw one. If you are experienced with cooking and preparing artichokes, use fresh artichokes in the same quantity as the canned.

PER SERVING Calories: 75; Total fat: 3g; Saturated fat: 0g; Carbohydrates: 11g; Fiber: 3g; Protein: 5g

SEASONED CARROT BATONS

SERVES 4 **PREP** 15 minutes **COOK** 20 minutes

The seasoning for this savory side tastes a little like ranch dressing without the creamy base. Use this versatile herb mixture for other dishes beyond carrots, such as chicken or pork. It keeps for up to one month in a sealed container if you want to double or triple the amounts. If you have leftover carrots, toss them in a kale or spinach smoothie for added flavor.

Vegan

2 tablespoons olive oil, plus more for greasing the baking sheet

1 teaspoon dried parsley

1 teaspoon garlic powder

¼ teaspoon onion powder

¼ teaspoon dried dill

Pinch sea salt

8 carrots, peeled and cut into ½-inch-wide and 3-inch-long sticks

1 tablespoon chopped fresh dill

1. Preheat the oven to 400°F.

2. Lightly grease a rimmed baking sheet with olive oil, and set it aside.

3. In a small bowl, stir together the parsley, garlic powder, onion powder, dill, and sea salt.

4. Spread the carrots on the baking sheet. Sprinkle with the seasoning mix and drizzle with the remaining 2 tablespoons of olive oil.

5. Roast the carrots for about 20 minutes, or until lightly caramelized and tender. Transfer to a serving bowl and garnish with the fresh dill.

PREPARATION TIP To reduce the chopping needed, purchase precut and peeled baby carrots or just cut full-size carrots into chunks or slices.

PER SERVING Calories: 115; Total fat: 7g; Saturated fat: 1g; Carbohydrates: 13g; Fiber: 3g; Protein: 1g

BLANCHED GREEN VEGGIES WITH RADISHES

SERVES 4   **PREP** 15 minutes   **COOK** 5 minutes

Radishes are most frequently seen in cold salads but they are equally delicious when warmed. This vibrant, pleasingly hot vegetable is only warmed rather than cooked, so don't be surprised at the crunch. This is an excellent accompaniment for a perfectly grilled chicken breast or snowy white, moist baked fish such as halibut.

Vegan

1½ tablespoons olive oil

1 pound asparagus spears, woody ends trimmed

½ pound green beans, trimmed

1 cup fava beans (fresh or frozen and thawed)

1 cup peas (fresh or frozen and thawed)

½ cup whole radishes, trimmed

1 tablespoon rice vinegar

Sea salt

Freshly ground black pepper

1. Place a large skillet over medium heat and add the olive oil.

2. Add the asparagus, green beans, fava beans, and peas. Sauté for about 5 minutes, or until crisp-tender.

3. Add the radishes and rice vinegar, or and toss to combine.

4. Season the veggies with sea salt and pepper and serve.

COOKING TIP Constantly toss the vegetables with tongs while cooking, or those at the bottom of the pile will overcook. For best results, use a wok so you can move most of the ingredients to the sides off the direct heat.

PER SERVING Calories: 247; Total fat: 6g; Saturated fat: 1g; Carbohydrates: 35g; Fiber: 16g; Protein: 15g

CARAMELIZED CELERIAC

SERVES 4 **PREP** 10 minutes **COOK** 20 minutes

Celeriac, or celery root, is a bulbous fresh-tasting vegetable that is about the size of a grapefruit. It is available year round but is in season between September and April. The reason this vegetable can be found year round is that it can be stored between 32°F and 41°F for up to eight months. If you want a different texture for this dish, mash the roasted celeriac with the maple syrup and lemon juice instead of serving it in chunks. If celeriac can't be found at your local grocery store, good substitutions are parsley root (which will have a stronger flavor) or chopped celery (for a milder flavor).

Vegan

2 celeriac, peeled and diced

1 tablespoon olive oil

½ teaspoon ground nutmeg

½ teaspoon ground cinnamon

⅛ teaspoon sea salt

2 tablespoons pure maple syrup

1 teaspoon freshly squeezed lemon juice

1. Preheat the oven to 400°F.

2. Line a rimmed baking sheet with aluminum foil.

3. In a large bowl, toss together the celeriac, olive oil, nutmeg, cinnamon, and sea salt.

4. Spread the celeriac on the prepared sheet and roast for 15 to 20 minutes, or until very tender and lightly caramelized.

5. Transfer the celeriac to a serving bowl. Add the maple syrup and lemon juice. Toss to coat and then serve.

INGREDIENT TIP Celeriac can be a tricky vegetable to buy because it is often a bit old and wizened by the time someone picks it up in the grocery store. Look for celeriac that feels slightly heavier than it looks, has no wet or soft spots, and has a smooth, pale skin.

SUBSTITUTION TIP If you can't find celeriac, use carrots, parsnips, squash, sweet potatoes, or turnips instead.

PER SERVING Calories: 157; Total fat: 4g; Saturated fat: 1g; Carbohydrates: 29g; Fiber: 4g; Protein: 4g

SLOW-ROASTED SWEET POTATOES

SERVES 4 **PREP** 10 minutes **COOK** 40 minutes

Sweet potatoes often get a bad reputation because they are frequently prepared with butter, cream, candied nuts, and even mini marshmallows. This vegetable, though, is actually a very healthy addition to any diet. Sweet potatoes are extremely high in vitamins A and C as well as an excellent source of manganese, copper, and beta-carotene. Including sweet potatoes regularly in your meals can help reduce inflammation in the body, improve digestion, and support the cardiovascular system.

Make Ahead

Vegan

Olive oil, for greasing the baking dish

3 sweet potatoes, peeled and cut into large chunks

1 tablespoon pure maple syrup

½ teaspoon ground allspice

½ teaspoon ground ginger

¼ teaspoon ground nutmeg

Pinch sea salt

½ cup unsweetened apple juice

1. Preheat the oven to 350°F.

2. Lightly grease an 8-by-8-inch baking dish with olive oil.

3. In a large bowl, toss the sweet potatoes, maple syrup, allspice, ginger, nutmeg, and sea salt until well mixed. Transfer the sweet potatoes to the prepared dish, and pour in the apple juice.

4. Cover the dish and bake the potatoes for about 40 minutes, or until very tender.

COOKING TIP These delectable potatoes can be cooked easily in a slow cooker. Place everything in the insert, cover, and cook for 8 hours on low or 4 hours on high heat.

PER SERVING Calories: 295; Total fat: 1g; Saturated fat: 0g; Carbohydrates: 70g; Fiber: 9g; Protein: 4g

SAUTÉED KALE WITH GARLIC

SERVES 4 **PREP** 15 minutes **COOK** 12 minutes

Being delicious does not mean a dish has to be complicated and ingredient packed. Simple sautéed greens can burst with flavor and look glorious on your plate next to almost anything. Kale is the perfect dark leafy green to toss with a little olive oil, vinegar, and garlic because it has an assertive earthy taste that holds its own with other flavors. Try different types of kale such as lacinato, Redbor, and curly kale to experience the variety of textures and colors available.

Vegan

1 tablespoon olive oil

3 garlic cloves, thinly sliced

8 cups chopped kale

1 tablespoon balsamic vinegar

½ teaspoon ground nutmeg

Sea salt

1. In a large skillet over medium heat, sauté the olive oil and garlic for about 4 minutes, or until the garlic is lightly caramelized and very fragrant.

2. Add the kale. Cover and sauté for about 5 minutes, or until the leaves have wilted.

3. Uncover and cook for about 3 minutes more until all the liquid has evaporated.

4. Stir in the balsamic vinegar, sprinkle with nutmeg, and season with sea salt.

SUBSTITUTION TIP Dark leafy greens are, as a group, one of the healthier ingredients in any diet, so feel free to swap the kale in this dish for spinach, beet greens, Swiss chard, or any other comparable choice. You might have a preference for a particular taste or texture other than kale.

PER SERVING Calories: 102; Total fat: 4g; Saturated fat: 1g; Carbohydrates: 15g; Fiber: 2g; Protein: 4g

BUCKWHEAT TABBOULEH

SERVES 4 **PREP** 15 minutes **COOK** 10 minutes

Tabbouleh is usually made into a cold salad rather than a warm side dish, but the ingredients are so similar that this variation works. The prominent herb in any tabbouleh is parsley because of its unique taste and wonderful health benefits. Parsley is extremely high in vitamin K: each serving of this dish contains about 125 percent of the recommended daily amount. Parsley is also a spectacular source of vitamins C and A, powerful disease-fighting antioxidants.

Make Ahead

Vegan

1 tablespoon olive oil

½ cup chopped red onion

2 teaspoons bottled minced garlic

2 cups cooked buckwheat

Juice of 1 lemon (3 tablespoons)

Zest of 1 lemon (optional)

½ cup chopped fresh parsley

¼ cup chopped fresh mint

Sea salt

1. Place a large skillet over medium-high heat and add the olive oil.

2. Add the red onion and garlic. Sauté for about 3 minutes, or until translucent.

3. Stir in the buckwheat, lemon juice, and lemon zest (if using). Sauté for about 5 minutes, or until heated through.

4. Stir in the parsley and mint. Sauté for 1 minute more.

5. Remove from the heat and season with sea salt.

PREPARATION TIP Buckwheat can be simmered in water in the same way you prepare pasta. Just drain off the excess water when the buckwheat is tender, and use it right away or refrigerate it for up to 3 days. Additionally, the herbs and onion can be chopped in a food processor to minimize prep work and chopping.

PER SERVING Calories: 184; Total fat: 5g; Saturated fat: 1g; Carbohydrates: 34g; Fiber: 5g; Protein: 6g

WILD RICE–CAULIFLOWER PILAF

SERVES 4   **PREP** 10 minutes   **COOK** 45 minutes

Wild rice is one of the most interesting looking and attractive ingredients you will find for a filling side dish. The glossy dark color contrasts dramatically with the bright orange and pale white of the vegetables. Do not overcook wild rice, because it becomes dull, falls apart, and is not as delicious. You will also find that perfectly cooked wild rice reheats easily and makes superior leftovers.

Make Ahead

1 tablespoon olive oil, plus more for greasing the baking dish

2 cups Herbed Chicken Bone Broth (page 76)

1 cup raw wild rice

2 stalks celery, chopped, or about ¾ to 1 cup precut packaged celery

1 sweet onion, chopped, or about 1 cup precut packaged onion

1 teaspoon bottled minced garlic

½ cauliflower head, chopped into small florets, or 2½ to 3 cups precut packaged florets

2 carrots, peeled, halved lengthwise, and sliced, or about 1 cup precut packaged carrots

1 teaspoon chopped fresh thyme

Sea salt

1. Preheat the oven to 350°F.

2. Lightly grease an 8-by-8-inch baking dish with olive oil and set it aside.

3. In a large saucepan over high heat, stir together the chicken broth and wild rice. Bring the mixture to a boil. Reduce the heat to low and simmer for about 30 minutes, or until the rice is tender.

4. While the rice cooks, place a large skillet over medium-high heat and add the remaining 1 tablespoon of olive oil.

5. Add the celery, onion, and garlic. Sauté for about 3 minutes, or until tender.

6. Add the cauliflower and carrots and sauté for 5 minutes. Remove the skillet from the heat and set it aside until the rice is done.

7. Transfer the cooked rice to the skillet. Stir in the thyme. Season with sea salt and spoon the mixture into the prepared dish.

8. Bake for about 15 minutes, or until the vegetables are tender.

INGREDIENT TIP Wild rice is an aquatic grass seed indigenous to freshwater lakes and rivers in Canada and some northern states in the United States. Make sure your rice package indicates it is 100 percent wild rice, because many products are blends of other grains.

PER SERVING Calories: 213; Total fat: 4g; Saturated fat: 1g; Carbohydrates: 38g; Fiber: 5g; Protein: 7g

VEGETABLE QUINOA

SERVES 4 **PREP** 15 minutes **COOK** 25 minutes plus 10 minutes resting

Asparagus is one of the loveliest vegetables, with its tightly bunched tips and slender stalks, especially in the spring when they are in season and incredibly tender. If you cannot find pencil-width asparagus, use a vegetable peeler to remove the woodier layers. Asparagus is a wonderful source of vitamin A and is considered to be an antioxidant and anti-inflammatory. Asparagus supports healthy vision, fights cancer, and supports the cardiovascular system.

Make Ahead

1 tablespoon olive oil

½ sweet onion, diced, or about ½ cup precut packaged onion

2 teaspoons bottled minced garlic

1 cup finely shredded cabbage

1 cup (2-inch) asparagus pieces

1 carrot, finely chopped, or about ½ cup precut packaged carrots

1 tablespoon freshly grated lemon zest (optional)

1 teaspoon ground cumin

¼ teaspoon ground nutmeg

2½ cups Herbed Chicken Bone Broth (page 76)

1 cup quinoa, rinsed well

Pinch sea salt

1 teaspoon chopped fresh thyme

1. Place a large saucepan over medium-high heat and add the olive oil.

2. Add the onion and garlic. Sauté for about 3 minutes, or until tender.

3. Add the cabbage, asparagus, carrot, lemon zest (if using), cumin, and nutmeg. Sauté for 2 minutes.

4. Stir in the chicken broth, quinoa, and sea salt. Bring the mixture to a boil. Reduce the heat to low, and simmer for about 20 minutes, or until the vegetables are tender and the liquid has been absorbed.

5. Remove the saucepan from the heat, cover, and let it sit for 10 minutes.

6. Fluff the quinoa with a fork and serve sprinkled with the thyme.

INGREDIENT TIP Rinse quinoa well before using because it has a soapy coating of saponins, which creates a bitter taste. Saponins can also be the cause of stomach issues for people who are sensitive to this phytochemical.

PER SERVING Calories: 222; Total fat: 7g; Saturated fat: 1g; Carbohydrates: 34g; Fiber: 5g; Protein: 8g

COCONUT-ALMOND BAKE

SERVES 4 **PREP** 10 minutes **COOK** 25 minutes

If you top each portion individually with scallions rather than garnish the entire serving bowl, you can enjoy leftovers of this side dish for breakfast. It is creamy and slightly sweet and can be reheated on the stove top with a little almond milk in a couple minutes. The onion and garlic are not overpowering, so you will not feel strange starting your day with a slightly savory porridge.

Make Ahead
Vegan

1 tablespoon olive oil

1 sweet onion, chopped, or about 1 cup precut packaged onion

1 tablespoon grated fresh ginger, or 1 teaspoon ground ginger

2 teaspoons bottled minced garlic

1 cup canned lite coconut milk

1 cup water

1 cup quinoa, rinsed well

¼ cup chopped toasted almonds

1 scallion, white and green parts, chopped

1. Place a large saucepan over medium-high heat and add the olive oil.

2. Add the onion, ginger, and garlic. Sauté for about 3 minutes, or until softened.

3. Stir in the coconut milk, water, and quinoa. Bring the mixture to a boil. Reduce the heat to low, cover, and simmer for about 20 minutes, or until the quinoa is tender and the liquid has been absorbed.

4. Stir in the almonds and serve topped with the scallions.

SUBSTITUTION TIP If tree nuts are a concern for you, omit the almonds. They add a little extra crunch and flavor, but the side dish is still delicious and satisfying without them.

PER SERVING Calories: 378; Total fat: 24g; Saturated fat: 14g; Carbohydrates: 36g; Fiber: 6g; Protein: 9g

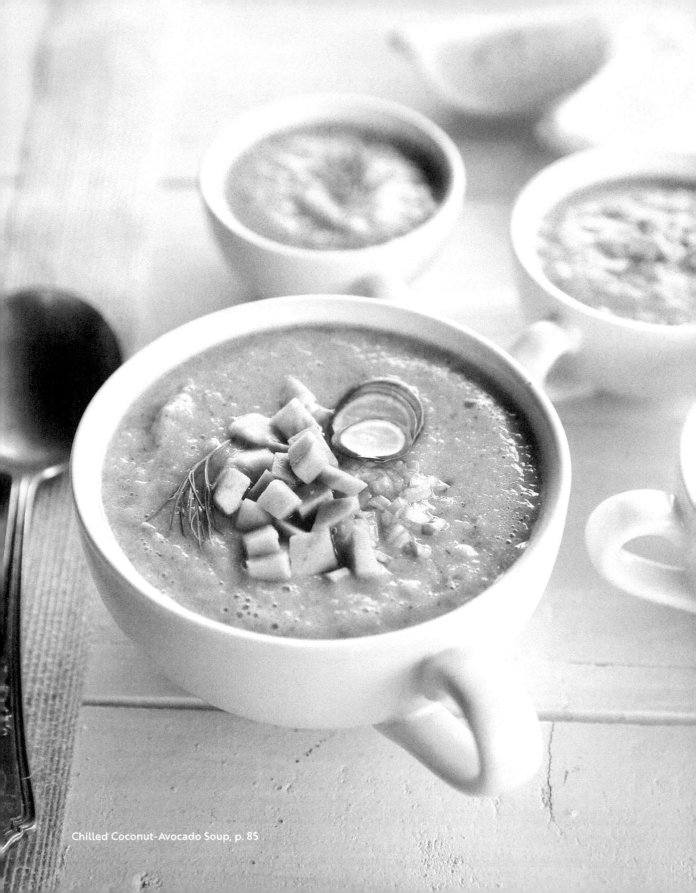

Chilled Coconut-Avocado Soup, p. 85

5

SOUPS

HERBED CHICKEN BONE BROTH

MAKES 8 to 10 cups **PREP** 10 minutes **COOK** 24 hours, 30 minutes

You might be wondering what the difference is between regular stock and bone broth because the ingredients look similar. Stock is simmered for only a moderate amount of time—about 6 hours—rather than the long-simmering bone broth. The goal of bone broth is to release the nutritious minerals, collagen, and amino acids from the bones, along with their gelatin. Consuming this product can help heal the gut, which can be very important when you are trying to follow a diet that addresses rheumatoid arthritis.

Make Ahead

2 chicken carcasses

3 tablespoons apple cider vinegar

2 carrots, washed and roughly chopped

2 stalks celery, quartered

1 sweet onion, peeled and quartered

4 garlic cloves, smashed

4 fresh thyme sprigs

2 fresh rosemary sprigs

2 bay leaves

1. Preheat the oven to 350°F.

2. Place the chicken carcasses in a baking pan and roast for 30 minutes. Transfer the carcasses to a large stockpot. Add enough cold water to cover the carcasses by 2 inches, and the cider vinegar. Place the stockpot over high heat and bring to a boil. Reduce the heat to low and gently simmer for 18 hours, stirring every few hours.

3. Add the carrots, celery, onion, garlic, thyme, rosemary, and bay leaves, and bring to a boil again. Reduce the heat to low and simmer the broth for 6 hours more, stirring several times.

4. Remove the pot from the heat and let the broth cool slightly.

5. With tongs, remove and discard any large bones from the pot. Strain the broth through a fine-mesh sieve and discard any solid bits.

6. Pour the chicken broth into sealable containers and let it cool completely.

7. Refrigerate the broth for up to 7 days, or freeze for up to 3 months.

SUBSTITUTION TIP Save chicken carcasses from previously roasted birds by placing them in the freezer after the meat is stripped off. If you use these "cooked" carcasses, skip the roasting in step 2.

PER SERVING Calories: 60; Total fat: 3g; Saturated fat: 1g; Carbohydrates: 0g; Fiber: 0g; Protein: 1g

BEEF BONE BROTH

MAKES 8 to 10 cups   **PREP** 10 minutes   **COOK** 24 hours, 30 minutes

If you have never made beef stock or broth before, you might be at a loss about where to find beef bones. This inexpensive ingredient has probably been sitting in the meat aisle next to the steaks and ground beef, but you never noticed it before. Beef bones can also be found at reputable butchers or behind the meat counter in your supermarket if you ask the butcher.

Make Ahead

2 pounds beef bones

3 tablespoons apple cider vinegar

2 carrots, washed and roughly chopped

2 stalks celery, roughly chopped

1 sweet onion, peeled and quartered

3 garlic cloves, smashed

1. Preheat the oven to 350°F.

2. Place the beef bones in a roasting pan and roast them for 30 minutes. Transfer the bones to a large stockpot and add enough cold water to cover them by 2 inches, and the cider vinegar. Place the stockpot over high heat and bring to a boil. Reduce the heat to low and simmer for 18 hours. Check the broth every 30 minutes for the first 2 hours for any impurities floating on the top. Skim off the impurities with a spoon.

3. Add the carrots, celery, onion, and garlic. Bring the liquid back to a boil. Simmer for 6 hours more.

4. Remove the pot from the heat and let the broth cool slightly.

5. With tongs, remove and discard any large bones from the pot. Strain the broth through a fine-mesh sieve and discard any solid bits.

6. Pour the broth into sealable containers and let it cool completely.

7. Refrigerate the broth for up to 7 days, or freeze for up to 3 months.

COOKING TIP For an even richer broth, roast the onion, carrots, celery, and garlic in the roasting pan with the bones and throw them in the stockpot right from the oven. The vegetables break down more in the water, but the lightly caramelized taste is oh so good.

PER SERVING Calories: 80; Total fat: 5g; Saturated fat: 1g; Carbs: 0g; Fiber: 0g; Protein: 4g

LUSCIOUS SWEET POTATO SOUP

SERVES 6   **PREP** 15 minutes   **COOK** 35 minutes

Sweet potatoes are not the only vegetable in this scrumptious soup that adds bright color—the carrots also create a warm orange hue. As with sweet potatoes, carrots are an outstanding source of beta-carotene, vitamins A and K, and fiber. Carrots can help reduce the risk of degenerative eye diseases such as glaucoma, support the immune system, and promote a healthy heart.

Make Ahead

1 tablespoon olive oil

1 sweet onion, chopped, or about 1 cup precut packaged onion

2 teaspoons grated fresh ginger

8 cups Herbed Chicken Bone Broth (page 76)

2 pounds sweet potatoes (about 4), peeled and diced, or 6 cups precut packaged sweet potatoes

1 carrot, diced, or ¾ cup precut packaged carrots

¼ cup pure maple syrup

1 teaspoon ground cinnamon

¼ teaspoon ground nutmeg

1 cup coconut cream, plus 1 tablespoon for garnish

Sea salt

1. Place a large stockpot over medium-high heat and add the olive oil.

2. Add the onion and ginger. Sauté for about 3 minutes, or until softened.

3. Stir in the chicken broth, sweet potatoes, carrot, maple syrup, cinnamon, and nutmeg. Bring the soup to a boil. Reduce the heat to low and simmer for about 30 minutes, or until the vegetables are tender.

4. Working in batches, purée the soup in a food processor until very smooth. Transfer the soup back to the pot.

5. Stir in the coconut cream and reheat the soup.

6. Season with sea salt, drizzle with coconut cream, garnish with a fresh herb of your choice, and serve.

VARIATION TIP Yams and sweet potatoes are often used interchangeably even though they are very different in taste and color. You can use yams in this soup for a change, but you might notice the finished dish is not as sweet.

PER SERVING Calories: 353; Total fat: 13g; Saturated fat: 9g; Carbohydrates: 58g; Fiber: 8g; Protein: 5g

CLASSIC FRENCH ONION SOUP

SERVES 4 **PREP** 15 minutes **COOK** 2 hours, 30 minutes

French onion soup is a culinary masterpiece that is often smothered in huge broth-sucking chunks of bread and a greasy topping of melted cheese. This unhealthy presentation completely masks the natural sweetness of caramelized onions and the richness of the beef broth. Onions are an incredibly healthy ingredient because they are packed with flavonoids, which help slow the destruction of the body's cells. Onions are the best source of a flavonoid called quercetin, which helps fight cancer and is very supportive of the cardiovascular system.

2 tablespoons olive oil

3 pounds sweet onions, halved and cut into ⅛-inch-thick slices (a mandoline or food processor slicing disc helps here)

2 teaspoons bottled minced garlic

½ cup dry sherry

8 cups Beef Bone Broth (page 78)

1 tablespoon chopped fresh thyme

Sea salt

Freshly ground black pepper

1. Place a large stockpot over low heat and add the olive oil.

2. Add the onions and garlic. Cover the pot and cook for 30 minutes, letting the juices purge from the onions. Stir occasionally.

3. Remove the lid. Continue to sauté the onions and garlic, stirring occasionally, for about 1 hour, 30 minutes, or until they are a deep caramel color.

4. Add the sherry and deglaze the pan, scraping up any browned bits from the bottom.

5. Increase the heat to medium. Stir in the beef broth and thyme. Bring the soup to a boil. Reduce the heat to low and simmer for about 30 minutes, or until the onions are tender.

6. Season with sea salt and pepper.

SUBSTITUTION TIP Sherry adds another layer of flavor to the onion soup, and the alcohol cooks out of the liquid. However, if you want to omit this ingredient, add ¼ cup balsamic vinegar instead.

PER SERVING Calories: 234; Total fat: 9g; Saturated fat: 2g; Carbohydrates: 33g; Fiber: 8g; Protein: 9g

CREAM OF BROCCOLI SOUP

SERVES 6 **PREP** 15 minutes **COOK** 35 minutes

Broccoli just looks like a happy, healthy ingredient with its lovely, almost frilly, florets and deep green color. It's usually a sure bet that vegetables as green as broccoli contain lots of a complex chemical called chlorophyll, which is crucial for photosynthesis in plants. Chlorophyll is also very beneficial for people because it cleanses the blood and boosts the ability of red blood cells to carry oxygen.

1 tablespoon olive oil

1 sweet onion, chopped, or about 1 cup precut packaged onion

2 teaspoons bottled minced garlic

8 cups Herbed Chicken Bone Broth (page 76)

3 heads broccoli, cut into florets, or 8 cups precut packaged florets

1 sweet potato, peeled and roughly chopped, or 1½ cups precut packaged sweet potatoes

1 teaspoon ground nutmeg

½ cup coconut cream

Sea salt

1. Place a large stockpot over medium-high heat, and add the olive oil.

2. Add the onion and garlic. Sauté for about 3 minutes, or until softened.

3. Stir in the chicken broth, broccoli, sweet potato, and nutmeg. Bring the soup to a boil. Reduce the heat to low and simmer for about 30 minutes, or until the vegetables are tender.

4. Working in batches, purée the soup in a food processor until smooth. Transfer the soup back to a pot.

5. Whisk in the coconut cream and season with sea salt.

COOKING TIP Use the broccoli stalks in the soup as well because they are full of flavor and nutritional benefits. Chop the stalks into ½-inch pieces and throw them in with the florets.

PER SERVING Calories: 197; Total fat: 10g; Saturated fat: 5g; Carbohydrates: 19g; Fiber: 6g; Protein: 12g

SUMMER VEGETABLE SOUP

SERVES 4   **PREP** 20 minutes   **COOK** 35 minutes

What would a summer soup be without lots of fresh basil? Basil is a hearty herb that features lovely dark green leaves and a slight licorice flavor. This pretty herb is very high in vitamin K, copper, manganese, magnesium, and flavonoids such as orientin and vicenin, which can fight inflammation in the body. Basil also supports the cardiovascular system and digestive system.

Vegan

1 tablespoon olive oil

2 stalks celery, chopped, or about ¾ to 1 cup precut packaged celery

1 sweet onion, chopped, or about 1 cup precut packaged onion

2 teaspoons bottled minced garlic

2 carrots, halved lengthwise and thinly sliced, or about 1 to 1½ cups precut packaged carrots

1 sweet potato, peeled and diced, or 1½ cups precut packaged sweet potatoes

8 cups low-sodium vegetable broth

2 cups (1-inch) green bean pieces

1 cup cauliflower florets

2 tablespoons chopped fresh basil

Sea salt

Freshly ground black pepper

1. In a large stockpot over medium-high heat, heat the olive oil.

2. Add the celery, onion, and garlic. Sauté for about 4 minutes, or until softened.

3. Add the carrots and sweet potato. Sauté for 3 minutes.

4. Stir in the vegetable broth. Bring the soup to a boil. Reduce the heat to low and simmer the soup for about 20 minutes, or until the vegetables are crisp-tender.

5. Stir in the green beans, cauliflower, and basil. Simmer for 5 minutes.

6. Season the soup with sea salt and pepper and serve.

VARIATION TIP Vegetable soups are wonderfully versatile, especially when they feature an assortment of veggies like this creation. Whatever is in your refrigerator and pantry can be used in this soup, so get creative and clean out your produce bins at the same time. If you would like to add more protein and having a vegan dish is not a concern, toss in some shredded chicken or cooked ground beef for added nutrients and flavor.

PER SERVING Calories: 140; Total fat: 4g; Saturated fat: 1g; Carbohydrates: 21g; Fiber: 7g; Protein: 4g

CURRIED CAULIFLOWER SOUP

SERVES 6 **PREP** 15 minutes **COOK** 40 minutes

Cruciferous vegetables, such as cauliflower, are a family that nutritionists recommend we consume every day because they are so nutritious. Cauliflower is a brilliant source of vitamins C and K, omega-3 fatty acids, and manganese, which is beneficial to the heart, brain, and digestive system. This warmly spiced soup would be perfect poured into a huge pottery mug and sipped on a cool autumn evening on a starlit patio.

1 tablespoon olive oil

1 sweet onion, chopped, or about 1 cup precut packaged onion

2 teaspoons bottled minced garlic

8 cups Herbed Chicken Bone Broth (page 76)

2 heads cauliflower, cut into small florets, or about 8 cups precut packaged florets, divided

1 tablespoon Mild Curry Powder (page 50)

1 cup coconut cream

Sea salt

2 tablespoons chopped fresh cilantro

1. Place a large stockpot over medium-high heat and add the olive oil.

2. Add the onion and garlic. Sauté for about 3 minutes, or until softened.

3. Stir in the chicken broth, three-fourths of the cauliflower florets, and the curry powder. Bring the soup to a boil. Reduce the heat to low and simmer for about 30 minutes, or until the cauliflower is tender.

4. While the soup simmers, blanch the remaining fourth of the cauliflower florets in boiling water for about 4 minutes, or until crisp-tender. Drain and set aside.

5. Working in batches, purée the soup in a food processor until smooth. Return the soup to the pot.

6. Stir in the coconut cream and reserved blanched cauliflower, and season the soup with sea salt.

7. Serve garnished with the cilantro.

COOKING TIP If you want to freeze this soup, leave out the coconut cream until you reheat it on the stove at a later time. This ensures a luscious, smooth texture.

PER SERVING Calories: 197; Total fat: 13g; Saturated fat: 9g; Carbohydrates: 11g; Fiber: 4g; Protein: 10g

CHILLED COCONUT-AVOCADO SOUP

SERVES 6   **PREP** 15 minutes plus 1 hour chilling

If the name of this recipe creates a vision of a pale pastel creamy concoction, you will be delighted by the festive green color of the actual soup. This is a chilled dish, so there is no slaving over the stove or trying to purée steaming hot ingredients in batches. You can garnish this soup with different vegetables or herbs, but the radishes add a lovely splash of color. The hint of lemon beautifully highlights the other flavors in this exotic creation.

Make Ahead

3 ripe avocados, peeled and pitted

¼ red onion, chopped, or about ¼ cup precut packaged onion

1 cup Herbed Chicken Bone Broth (page 76)

1 tablespoon freshly squeezed lemon juice

1 garlic clove, crushed

1 teaspoon grated fresh ginger

½ teaspoon chopped fresh dill, plus fresh dill sprigs for garnish

2 cups canned full-fat coconut milk

Sea salt

Freshly ground black pepper

Sliced radishes, for garnish

1. Coarsely chop three of the four avocado halves. Dice the remaining half and set it aside for garnish.

2. In a food processor, combine the chopped avocado, onion, chicken broth, lemon juice, garlic, ginger, and chopped dill. Purée until very smooth. Transfer the avocado soup to a lidded container.

3. Whisk in the coconut milk.

4. Season with sea salt and pepper. Chill the soup for at least 1 hour.

5. Garnish with the diced avocado, radishes, and dill sprigs just before serving.

INGREDIENT TIP Coconut milk can be found in the dairy section and the organic or ethnic sections of the grocery store, depending on which product you need for a recipe. Make sure you use thick, luscious, canned coconut milk rather than the watery coconut drink in the big cartons, or the taste and texture of the dish will be compromised.

PER SERVING Calories: 395; Total fat: 39g; Saturated fat: 21g; Carbohydrates: 14g; Fiber: 9g; Protein: 4g

VEGETABLE NOODLE BOWL

SERVES 4 **PREP** 20 minutes **COOK** 20 minutes

Coconut aminos is one of the best substitutions for soy sauce, and it is lower in sodium. Like the name suggests, coconut aminos is made from coconut sap. It is an excellent source of amino acids, potassium, and vitamin C. You can find it in most supermarkets right next to the soy sauce, or in the organic section. Coconut aminos can decrease inflammation in the body, improve blood pressure, and help stabilize blood sugar. For a protein boost, add some shredded cooked chicken or ground beef to this bowl if you do not need a vegetarian dish.

Make Ahead

Vegetarian

3 cups canned lite coconut milk

1 cup low-sodium vegetable broth

1 tablespoon coconut aminos

1 tablespoon raw honey

3 garlic cloves

¼ sweet onion, or about ¼ cup precut packaged onion

1 (2-inch) piece fresh ginger, peeled

Juice of 1 lime (1 or 2 tablespoons)

Zest of 1 lime (optional)

1 large carrot, julienned or spiralized

1 parsnip, julienned or spiralized

1 cup shredded bok choy

1 cup bean sprouts

2 tablespoons chopped fresh cilantro

1. In a blender, combine the coconut milk, vegetable broth, coconut aminos, honey, garlic, onion, ginger, lime juice (if using), and lime zest. Pulse until puréed. Pour the mixture into a large saucepan and bring to a boil over high heat. Reduce the heat to low and simmer for 15 minutes.

2. Stir in the carrot, parsnip, bok choy, and bean sprouts. Simmer for about 4 minutes, or until the vegetables are tender.

3. Serve topped with the cilantro.

COOKING TIP The julienned or spiralized vegetables will stay fresh in the refrigerator in a sealed container for up to 3 days. You can prep almost all the ingredients for this tempting dish ahead and throw it together in less than 30 minutes.

PER SERVING Calories: 183; Total fat: 10g; Saturated fat: 9g; Carbohydrates: 25g; Fiber: 3g; Protein: 6g

SOUTHWEST FISH SOUP

SERVES 6   **PREP** 15 minutes   **COOK** 25 minutes

You might notice when you read the ingredients that this is not strictly a fish soup as it also contains shrimp. That flexibility is one of the reasons fish soup is so popular in so many cultures: any ingredient works in the mix. This version uses chicken bone broth as a base, but you can certainly use a good-quality purchased fish broth or, even better, a homemade fish stock.

1 tablespoon olive oil

1 sweet onion, chopped, or about 1 cup precut packaged onion

2 stalks celery, chopped, or about ¾ to 1 cup precut packaged celery

2 teaspoons bottled minced garlic

6 cups Herbed Chicken Bone Broth (page 76)

2 cups cubed sweet potato

2 carrots, diced, or about 1½ cups precut packaged carrots

½ teaspoon ground cumin

½ teaspoon ground coriander

1 pound haddock, cut into 1-inch pieces

½ pound peeled and deveined shrimp, chopped

1 cup fresh spinach

2 tablespoons chopped fresh cilantro

1. Place a large stockpot over medium-high heat and add the olive oil.

2. Add the onion, celery, and garlic. Sauté for about 3 minutes, or until softened.

3. Stir in the chicken broth, sweet potato, carrots, cumin, and coriander. Bring the soup to a boil. Reduce the heat to low and simmer for about 10 minutes, or until the vegetables are tender.

4. Stir in the haddock and shrimp. Simmer for 10 minutes more.

5. Stir in the spinach and simmer for 2 minutes.

6. Serve the soup topped with the cilantro.

SUBSTITUTION TIP Any firm-fleshed fish can be added to this soup instead of haddock; just avoid delicate fish such as sole because it will break apart completely. If you need to omit the shrimp due to allergies, increase the fish by ½ pound to make up the portion size.

PER SERVING Calories: 255; Total fat: 8g; Saturated fat: 1g; Carbohydrates: 20g; Fiber: 3g; Protein: 26g

CHICKEN FENNEL SOUP

SERVES 4 **PREP** 20 minutes **COOK** 45 minutes

Cabbage provides a great deal of the bulk in this hearty soup, and each portion has a substantial amount of healthy fiber. Cabbage is a cruciferous vegetable, like cauliflower and broccoli, so it is very heart-friendly and reduces the risk of cancer. Cruciferous vegetables are also known to have goitrogenic properties, which means they can interfere with iodine uptake in the body, affecting thyroid function. The amount of cabbage in this soup is not detrimental, but if you have thyroid issues it is a good idea not to go overboard on cruciferous vegetables at every meal.

1 tablespoon olive oil

1 sweet onion, chopped, or about 1 cup precut packaged onion

2 teaspoons bottled minced garlic

3 cups shredded fennel

3 cups shredded green cabbage, or packaged shredded cabbage (see Tip)

2 carrots, chopped, or about 1 cup precut packaged carrots

8 cups Herbed Chicken Bone Broth (page 76)

2 teaspoons chopped fresh thyme

2 cups chopped cooked chicken breast

Pinch sea salt

1. Place a large stockpot over medium-high heat and add the olive oil.

2. Add the onion and garlic. Sauté for about 3 minutes, or until the onion is translucent.

3. Stir in the fennel, cabbage, and carrots. Sauté for about 5 minutes, or until the vegetables have softened.

4. Stir in the chicken broth and thyme. Bring the soup to a boil. Reduce the heat to low and simmer for about 30 minutes, or until the vegetables are tender.

5. Add the chicken and sea salt. Simmer for about 5 minutes, or until the chicken is heated through.

INGREDIENT TIP Packaged coleslaw mixes with cabbage and carrot or one featuring shredded broccoli stalks can be used if it is more convenient for you. Just check the date on the bag to ensure it is fresh.

PER SERVING Calories: 255; Total fat: 10g; Saturated fat: 2g; Carbohydrates: 16g; Fiber: 5g; Protein: 25g

BEEF AND VEGETABLE SOUP

SERVES 6   **PREP** 20 minutes   **COOK** 1 hour

Beef soups and stews are a staple in the cold-weather months; there is something stick-to-your-ribs about flavorsome beefy broth and chunks of meat and vegetables. The best part about them is that they help stretch your grocery dollars by using cheaper cuts of beef. Lean cuts of meat that grill up tough because of their lack of fat contain connective tissue called collagen that breaks down when simmered for a long time. This breaking down of tissue creates delectably tender meat chunks that are perfect in this soup.

2 tablespoons olive oil, divided

1 pound beef chuck roast, cut into ½-inch chunks

1 onion, chopped, or about 1 cup precut packaged onion

2 teaspoons bottled minced garlic

8 cups Beef Bone Broth (page 78)

2 carrots, diced, or about 1½ cups precut packaged carrots

2 turnips, peeled and diced, or 1½ cups precut packaged turnips

1 sweet potato, peeled and diced, or 1½ cups precut packaged sweet potatoes

2 bay leaves

2 cups frozen peas

2 teaspoons chopped fresh thyme

1 teaspoon chopped fresh parsley

Sea salt

Freshly ground black pepper

1. Place a large stockpot over medium-high heat and add 1 tablespoon of olive oil.

2. Add the beef in batches and brown, about 10 minutes total. Transfer the beef to a plate. Return the pot to the heat.

3. Add the remaining 1 tablespoon of olive oil to the pot along with the onion and garlic. Sauté for about 3 minutes, or until softened.

4. Stir in the beef broth, carrots, turnips, sweet potato, bay leaves, and the browned beef along with any accumulated juices on the plate. Bring to a boil. Reduce the heat to low and simmer the soup for about 45 minutes, or until the vegetables and beef are tender.

5. Remove and discard the bay leaves.

6. Stir in the peas, thyme, and parsley. Simmer for 4 minutes.

7. Season the soup with sea salt and pepper.

VARIATION TIP Pork, lamb, or venison makes a tasty soup in place of beef if you want a differently flavored soup. If you are adventurous, try bison or bear instead, if it is available where you live—the unique rich flavor is exceptional.

PER SERVING Calories: 452; Total fat: 28g; Saturated fat: 10g; Carbohydrates: 19g; Fiber: 5g; Protein: 30g

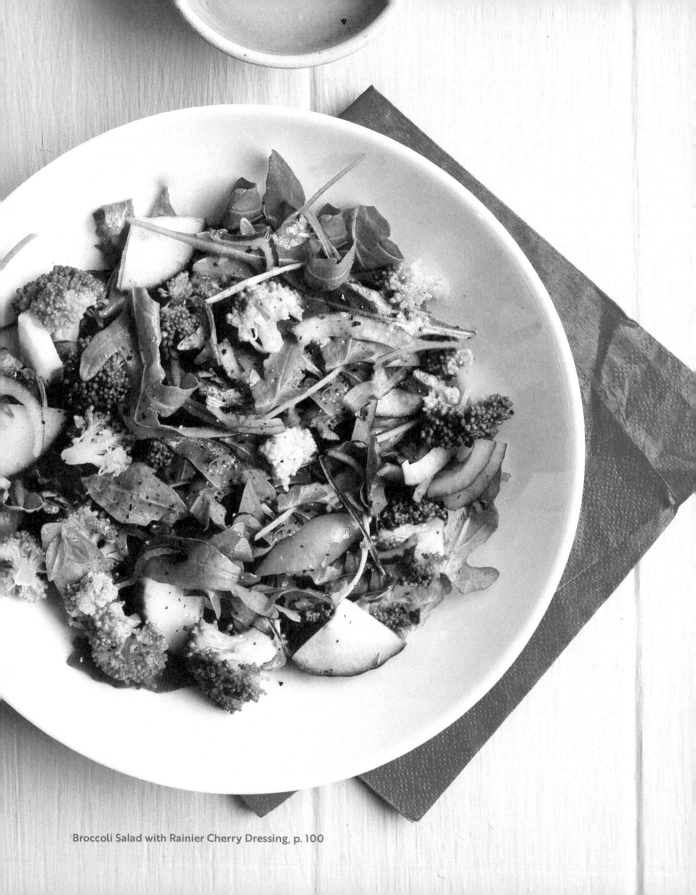

Broccoli Salad with Rainier Cherry Dressing, p. 100

6

SALADS

GREEN MANGO SLAW WITH CASHEWS

SERVES 4 **PREP** 35 minutes

Cashews are not actually nuts. This rich golden treat is the seed found at the bottom of the cashew apple. Cashews are a tremendous source of oleic acid—a monounsaturated fatty acid that is great for heart health and beneficial for those with diabetes. Despite being so high in oleic acid, cashews are lower in fat, on the whole, than other ingredients classed as nuts.

Make Ahead

Vegan

FOR THE DRESSING

1 cup canned lite coconut milk

2 tablespoons freshly squeezed lime juice

2 tablespoons almond butter

1 teaspoon grated fresh ginger

1 teaspoon Mild Curry Powder (page 50)

FOR THE SALAD

3 cups fresh spinach

2 green mangos, peeled, pitted, and julienned

1 jicama, shredded

1 carrot, shredded, or ½ cup preshredded packaged carrots

1 scallion, white and green parts, julienned

2 tablespoons chopped fresh cilantro

¼ cup chopped cashews, for garnish

TO MAKE THE DRESSING

In a small bowl, whisk the coconut milk, lime juice, almond butter, ginger, and curry powder until well blended. Set it aside.

TO MAKE THE SALAD

1. In a large bowl, toss together the spinach, mangos, jicama, carrot, and scallion.

2. Add the dressing and toss to coat.

3. Serve topped with the cilantro and cashews.

SUBSTITUTION TIP Omit the cashews as a garnish if tree nuts are a concern. For a little satisfying crunch, top the salad with the same quantity of pumpkin seeds instead.

INGREDIENT TIP If you are new to green mango, it's easy to work with. Simply peel it with a vegetable peeler and shred or julienne as needed for the recipe.

PER SERVING Calories: 415; Total fat: 24g; Saturated fat: 14g; Carbohydrates: 50g; Fiber: 14g; Protein: 8g

WATERMELON-CUCUMBER SALAD

SERVES 4 **PREP** 25 minutes

This succulent salad is so juicy and fresh, and the colorful presentation, featuring deep pink, pale green, bright green, and yellow, is stunning. Plus, the assortment of colors indicates lots of antioxidants. Watermelon is an excellent source of the antioxidant lycopene, which can reduce blood pressure by improving blood flow. Watermelon is also high in citrulline, an amino acid that supports the cardiovascular system.

Make Ahead
Vegetarian

FOR THE DRESSING

½ cup olive oil

¼ cup apple cider vinegar

2 tablespoons raw honey

1 teaspoon freshly grated lemon zest (optional)

Pinch sea salt

FOR THE SALAD

4 cups (½-inch) watermelon cubes

1 English cucumber, cut into ½-inch cubes

1 cup halved snow peas

1 scallion, white and green parts, chopped

2 cups shredded kale

1 tablespoon chopped fresh cilantro

TO MAKE THE DRESSING

In a small bowl, whisk the olive oil, cider vinegar, honey, and lemon zest (if using). Season with sea salt and set it aside.

TO MAKE THE SALAD

1. In a large bowl, toss together the watermelon, cucumber, snow peas, scallion, and dressing.

2. Divide the kale among four plates and top with the watermelon mixture.

3. Serve garnished with the cilantro.

COOKING TIP Try to leave some of the watermelon's pale green inner rind on the cubes because it is visually stunning and there is lots of nutrition packed in this underutilized area of the melon. The inner rind contains more citrulline than the pink part and is high in chlorophyll.

PER SERVING Calories: 353; Total fat: 26g; Saturated fat: 4g; Carbohydrates: 30g; Fiber: 3g; Protein: 4g

MASSAGED SWISS CHARD SALAD WITH CHOPPED EGG

SERVES 4　**PREP** 25 minutes

Dark leafy greens, in general, are packed with phytonutrients, fiber, vitamin K, B vitamins, and magnesium. Swiss chard is no exception. Chard can help slow the absorption of glucose in the body, so you will not experience a sugar rush if you enjoy this salad for lunch. This pretty green vegetable also contains a plethora of antioxidants, so it is extremely effective at fighting inflammation in the body.

Vegetarian

FOR THE DRESSING

¼ cup olive oil

3 tablespoons freshly squeezed lemon juice

2 teaspoons raw honey

1 teaspoon Dijon mustard

Sea salt

FOR THE SALAD

5 cups chopped Swiss chard

3 large hardboiled eggs, peeled and chopped

1 English cucumber, diced

½ cup sliced radishes

½ cup chopped pecans

FOR THE DRESSING

In a small bowl, whisk the olive oil, lemon juice, honey, and mustard. Season with salt and set it aside.

FOR THE SALAD

1. In a large bowl, toss the Swiss chard and dressing together for about 4 minutes, or until the greens start to soften. Divide the greens evenly among four plates.

2. Top each salad with egg, cucumber, radishes, and pecans.

SUBSTITUTION TIP If you are sensitive to eggs, omit them—the salad will still be delicious. Add a little chopped cooked chicken to increase the protein, if desired.

PER SERVING Calories: 241; Total fat: 21g; Saturated fat: 3g; Carbohydrates: 9g; Fiber: 2g; Protein: 7g

COCONUT FRUIT SALAD

SERVES 4   **PREP** 30 minutes

Although every ingredient in this sweet fruity salad is colorful and fresh, the strawberries take center stage with their heady fragrance and vibrant color. Strawberries are very high in beta-carotene, vitamin C, iron, and potassium. This combination of nutrients cuts the risk of cardiovascular disease, boosts the immune system, fights cancer, and stabilizes blood sugar. For the best flavor, look for in-season berries rather than imported products.

Make Ahead

Vegan

FOR THE DRESSING

¾ cup canned lite coconut milk

2 tablespoons almond butter

2 tablespoons freshly squeezed lime juice

FOR THE SALAD

6 cups mixed greens

½ pineapple, peeled, cored, and diced, or 3 cups precut packaged pineapple

1 mango, peeled, pitted, and diced, or 2 cups frozen chunks, thawed

1 cup quartered fresh strawberries

1 cup (1-inch) green bean pieces

½ cup shredded unsweetened coconut

1 tablespoon chopped fresh basil

TO MAKE THE DRESSING

In a small bowl, whisk the coconut milk, almond butter, and lime juice until smooth. Set it aside.

TO MAKE THE SALAD

1. In a large bowl, toss the mixed greens with three-fourths of the dressing. Arrange the salad on four plates.

2. In the same bowl, toss the pineapple, mango, strawberries, and green beans with the remaining fourth of the dressing.

3. Top each salad with the fruit and vegetable mixture and serve garnished with the coconut and basil.

INGREDIENT TIP For a sublime treat, crack a fresh coconut and grate the snowy flesh for this salad rather than using packaged dried shredded coconut. Reserve the coconut water for another recipe.

PER SERVING Calories: 311; Total fat: 19g; Saturated fat: 13g; Carbohydrates: 36g; Fiber: 7g; Protein: 5g

GRAPEFRUIT-AVOCADO SALAD

SERVES 4 **PREP** 20 minutes

Grapefruit is often a healthy choice for a balanced breakfast, but this sweet fruit is also extraordinary as a nutritious salad ingredient. Red grapefruit is recommended for this dish because of its luscious color, sweetness, and lycopene content. Lycopene is a phyto-nutrient that can help reduce the risk of cancer and cardiovascular disease. If you cannot find good-quality Ruby Red grapefruits, substitute the white variety.

Vegetarian

FOR THE DRESSING

½ avocado, peeled and pitted

¼ cup freshly squeezed lemon juice

2 tablespoons raw honey

Pinch sea salt

Water, for thinning the dressing

FOR THE SALAD

4 cups fresh spinach

1 Ruby Red grapefruit, peeled, sectioned, and cut into chunks

¼ cup sliced radishes

¼ cup roasted sunflower seeds

¼ cup dried cranberries

TO MAKE THE DRESSING

1. In a blender, combine the avocado, lemon juice, honey, and sea salt. Pulse until very smooth.

2. Add enough water to reach your desired consistency and set the dressing aside.

TO MAKE THE SALAD

1. In a large bowl toss the spinach with half the dressing. Divide the dressed spinach among four plates.

2. Top each with grapefruit, radishes, sunflower seeds, and cranberries.

3. Drizzle the remaining half of the dressing over the salads and serve.

COOKING TIP The lemon juice in the dressing ensures the avocado does not oxidize into an unsightly gray color. This creamy dressing keeps in the refrigerator for up to 4 days if you want to make it ahead.

PER SERVING Calories: 126; Total fat: 7g; Saturated fat: 1g; Carbohydrates: 16g; Fiber: 3g; Protein: 2g

SHREDDED ROOT VEGETABLE SALAD

SERVES 4 **PREP** 25 minutes

If you are a fan of coleslaw in all its variations, this salad might become a new favorite. There is not a bit of cabbage in sight, the dressing is not the usual mayonnaise-based mixture, and the diverse shredded vegetables are a delight to the eye and palate. Radish adds a dazzling hint of vibrant red and satisfying heat that combines beautifully with the subtle anise flavor of the fennel.

Make Ahead

Vegan

FOR THE DRESSING

¼ cup olive oil

3 tablespoons pure maple syrup

2 tablespoons apple cider vinegar

1 teaspoon grated fresh ginger

Sea salt

FOR THE SLAW

1 jicama, or 2 parsnips (see Tip), peeled and shredded

2 carrots, shredded, or 1 cup preshredded packaged carrots

½ celeriac, peeled and shredded

¼ fennel bulb, shredded

5 radishes, shredded

2 scallions, white and green parts, peeled and thinly sliced

½ cup pumpkin seeds, roasted

TO MAKE THE DRESSING

In a small bowl, whisk the olive oil, maple syrup, cider vinegar, and ginger until well blended. Season with sea salt and set it aside.

TO MAKE THE SLAW

1. In a large bowl, toss together the jicama, carrots, celeriac, fennel, radishes, and scallions.

2. Add the dressing and toss to coat.

3. Top the slaw with the pumpkin seeds and serve.

SUBSTITUTION TIP Jicama is not an unusual vegetable but it is sometimes absent in the produce section of the supermarket. If you cannot find jicama, use 2 medium parsnips instead. Likewise, if celeriac can't be found at your local grocery store, good substitutions are parsley root (which will have a stronger flavor) or chopped celery (for a milder flavor).

PER SERVING Calories: 343; Total fat: 21g; Saturated fat: 3g; Carbohydrates: 36g; Fiber: 11g; Protein: 7g

ARTICHOKE-ALMOND SALAD

SERVES 4 **PREP** 25 minutes

Supermarket shelves display several types of artichoke products such as chopped, quartered, whole, and those packed in water, oil, or seasoned vinegars. Water-packed artichokes add fewer calories than other varieties, which can be important if you are trying to lose weight. Artichokes are a stellar source of fiber and a great source of B vitamins, copper, calcium, and antioxidants. Artichokes can reduce the risk of cancer, promote liver health, and help reduce cholesterol.

Make Ahead

Vegan

2 cups cooked quinoa

2 (15-ounce) cans water-packed artichoke hearts, drained

1 cup chopped kale

½ cup chopped red onion

½ cup chopped almonds

3 tablespoons finely chopped fresh parsley

Juice of 1 lemon (or 3 tablespoons)

Zest of 1 lemon (optional)

2 tablespoons olive oil

1 tablespoon balsamic vinegar

1 teaspoon bottled minced garlic

Sea salt

1. In a large bowl, toss together the quinoa, artichoke hearts, kale, red onion, almonds, parsley, lemon juice, lemon zest (if using), olive oil, balsamic vinegar, and garlic until well mixed.

2. Season with sea salt and serve.

VARIATION TIP Substitute 1 tablespoon of sesame oil for 1 tablespoon of olive oil, and use golden toasted sesame seeds instead of almonds for an Asian-inspired salad. If you want to further follow this culinary theme, use gluten-free rice vinegar in place of the balsamic vinegar and garnish with julienned snow peas.

PER SERVING Calories: 402; Total fat: 16g; Saturated fat: 2g; Carbohydrates: 56g; Fiber: 17g; Protein: 16g

MINT-MELON SALAD

SERVES 4   **PREP** 20 minutes

Cantaloupe is one of the main components of this summer salad and, as you might have guessed by its sunny color, is very high in beta-carotene and vitamins A and C. You may have enjoyed juicy chunks of this melon before, but the fact that the seeds are edible and a stellar source of omega-3 fatty acids might surprise you. Rinse the seeds thoroughly after you remove them from the melon, pat them dry, and toast them in a 200°F oven for about 15 minutes, or until crunchy.

Make Ahead

Vegan

FOR THE DRESSING

3 tablespoons olive oil

2 tablespoons red wine vinegar

Sea salt

FOR THE SALAD

1 honeydew melon, rind removed, flesh cut into 1-inch cubes

½ cantaloupe, rind removed, flesh cut into 1-inch cubes

3 stalks celery, sliced, or about 1 to 1½ cups precut packaged celery

½ red onion, thinly sliced

¼ cup chopped fresh mint

TO MAKE THE DRESSING

In a small bowl, whisk the olive oil and red wine vinegar. Season with sea salt and set it aside.

TO MAKE THE SALAD

1. In a large bowl, combine the honeydew, cantaloupe, celery, red onion, and mint.

2. Add the dressing and toss to combine.

INGREDIENT TIP Mint comes in many varieties, although you will see spearmint or peppermint in most grocery stores. If you have a green thumb, grow a batch of pineapple or chocolate mint to use in this refreshing dressing.

PER SERVING Calories: 223; Total fat: 11g; Saturated fat: 2g; Carbohydrates: 32g; Fiber: 4g; Protein: 2g

BROCCOLI SALAD WITH RAINIER CHERRY DRESSING

SERVES 4 **PREP** 25 minutes

Rainer cherries are sweet, thick skinned, and creamy-white fleshed. This type of cherry is more expensive than regular black or red cherries, but they are worth every penny. Rainer cherries are in season in late June or early July, so make this salad at that time for the best results. You can use regular cherries if the premium cherries are not available.

Make Ahead

Vegetarian

FOR THE DRESSING

½ cup Rainier cherries, pitted

¼ cup olive oil

2 tablespoons freshly squeezed lemon juice

2 tablespoons raw honey

1 teaspoon chopped fresh basil

Pinch sea salt

FOR THE SALAD

4 cups broccoli florets, lightly blanched

2 cups mixed greens

1 cup snow peas

½ English cucumber, quartered lengthwise and sliced

½ red onion, thinly sliced

TO MAKE THE DRESSING

In a blender, combine the cherries, olive oil, lemon juice, honey, and basil. Pulse until smooth. Season with sea salt and set it aside.

TO MAKE THE SALAD

In a large bowl, toss the broccoli, greens, snow peas, cucumber, and red onion with the dressing to coat.

COOKING TIP Since the cherries in the dressing are puréed, it is okay to cut the pits out with a sharp paring knife, or purchase an inexpensive cherry pitter (found in most kitchen stores) to make the job neat and quick.

PER SERVING Calories: 189; Total fat: 13g; Saturated fat: 2g; Carbohydrates: 18g; Fiber: 3g; Protein: 3g

TURKEY-PECAN SALAD

SERVES 4 **PREP** 20 minutes

Turkey often is enjoyed only at big holiday dinners, and this flavorsome salad is a fabulous way to use up the piles of leftover turkey meat, both dark and white. Turkey is extremely high in protein—more than 30 grams per 4-ounce portion—so it can help stabilize post-meal blood sugar. Including turkey in your diet can also reduce your risk of cancer and support healthy nerve function.

FOR THE DRESSING

¼ cup olive oil

2 tablespoons balsamic vinegar

2 teaspoons whole-grain Dijon mustard

1 teaspoon chopped fresh thyme

Sea salt

FOR THE SALAD

4 cups mixed greens

1 cup arugula

½ red onion, thinly sliced

16 ounces cooked turkey breast, chopped

3 apricots, pitted and each fruit cut into 8 pieces

½ cup chopped pecans

TO MAKE THE DRESSING

In a small bowl, whisk the olive oil, balsamic vinegar, mustard, and thyme. Season with sea salt and set it aside.

TO MAKE THE SALAD

1. In a large bowl, toss together the mixed greens, arugula, and red onion with three-fourths of the dressing. Arrange the dressed salad on a serving platter.

2. Top the greens with the turkey, apricots, and pecans.

3. Drizzle with the remaining fourth of the dressing and serve.

SUBSTITUTION TIP Although they are in the title of this recipe, the pecans can be left out if allergies are a concern. A little extra crunch and richness of flavor can be added by using roasted sunflower seeds instead of the nuts.

PER SERVING Calories: 305; Total fat: 20g; Saturated fat: 3g; Carbohydrates: 12g; Fiber: 2g; Protein: 21g

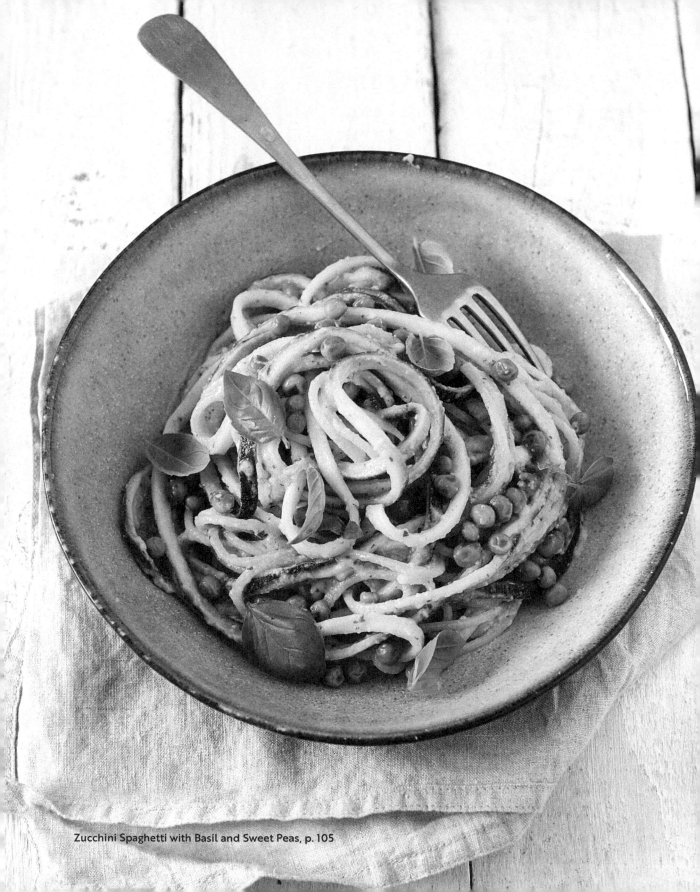

Zucchini Spaghetti with Basil and Sweet Peas, p. 105

7

VEGETARIAN & VEGAN

MUSHROOM EGG FOO YOUNG

SERVES 2 **PREP** 10 minutes **COOK** 20 minutes

Wild mushrooms include many delightfully earthy varieties such as shiitake, oyster, porto-bello, enoki, and cremini. Mushrooms are the only vegetable that contains vitamin D. They can support the immune system and cut the risk of cancer, arthritis, and cardiovascular disease. If you use portobello mushrooms, scoop out the black gills before adding them to the egg foo young or it will look gray.

Vegetarian

1 tablespoon olive oil

1 cup sliced wild mushrooms

1 teaspoon bottled minced garlic

2 cups bean sprouts

2 scallions, white and green parts, chopped

6 eggs

¼ teaspoon sea salt

1 tablespoon chopped fresh cilantro

1. Place a large skillet or wok over medium heat and add the olive oil.

2. Add the mushrooms and garlic. Sauté for about 4 minutes, or until softened.

3. Add the bean sprouts and scallions. Sauté for 5 minutes, spreading the vegetables out in the skillet.

4. In a small bowl, beat the eggs and sea salt. Pour the eggs over the vegetables in the skillet, shaking so the egg seeps through the vegetables. Cook for about 5 minutes, or until the eggs are set on the bottom.

5. Cut the omelet into quarters and flip them over. Cook the egg foo young for about 3 minutes, or until the omelet is completely cooked through.

6. Serve two pieces per person.

VARIATION TIP There is very little you can't put into egg foo young, even a vegetarian version. So try different vegetables depending on your palate. Celery, carrot, peas, bok choy, and asparagus tips would all be perfectly delicious when combined with the egg and bean sprouts base.

PER SERVING (2 pieces) Calories: 345; Total fat: 23g; Saturated fat: 6g; Carbohydrates: 12g; Fiber: 1g; Protein: 28g

ZUCCHINI SPAGHETTI WITH BASIL AND SWEET PEAS

SERVES 4 **PREP** 15 minutes

Spiralizers have become a must-have kitchen tool because many people follow various diets that do not allow standard pasta. These charming vegetable noodles can be served with an assortment of sauces and accompaniments. Simple fresh pesto and sweet peas create a dish that can go from refrigerator to table in about 15 minutes, leaving more time to enjoy the meal.

Make Ahead

Vegan

1 cup packed fresh basil leaves, plus more for garnish

1 cup packed fresh oregano leaves

½ cup almonds

2 teaspoons bottled minced garlic

Juice of 1 lemon (or 3 tablespoons)

Zest of 1 lemon (optional)

Pinch sea salt

Pinch freshly ground black pepper

¼ cup olive oil

2 large green zucchini, julienned or spiralized

1 cup peas (fresh or frozen and thawed)

1. In a food processor, combine the basil, oregano, almonds, garlic, lemon juice, lemon zest (if using), sea salt, and pepper. Pulse until very finely chopped.

2. While the processor is running, add the olive oil in a thin stream until a thick paste forms.

3. In a bowl, combine the zucchini noodles and peas. Add the pesto, 1 tablespoon at a time, until you have the desired flavor. Serve immediately, garnished with basil leaves.

4. Refrigerate any leftover pesto in a sealed container for up to 2 weeks.

COOKING TIP Depending on the length of the zucchini you use, you might want to snip the vegetable noodles into manageable lengths. With larger vegetables, the noodles can come out of the spiralizer in strands reaching several feet in length.

PER SERVING Calories: 280; Total fat: 21g; Saturated fat: 3g; Carbohydrates: 23g; Fiber: 12g; Protein: 8g

PAPAYA RICE BOWL

SERVES 4 **PREP** 20 minutes **COOK** 45 minutes

In the produce section of your local grocery store, you may have mistaken jicama for a very big potato, which would not be surprising because it is a root vegetable. After you remove the thick, almost fibrous skin, the white, crisp, juicy flesh might remind you of Asian pears. If you can find only a very large vegetable, use the extra jicama in smoothies, chopped in salsa, or as a delightful snack.

Make Ahead

Vegetarian

FOR THE SAUCE

2 tablespoons olive oil

Juice of ¼ lemon (about 1 tablespoon)

1 tablespoon raw honey

2 teaspoons chopped fresh basil

Sea salt

FOR THE RICE

1½ cups wild rice

2 cups shredded cabbage

2 papayas, peeled, seeded, and diced, or about 4 cups frozen (thawed) chunks

1 jicama, peeled and shredded

1 cup snow peas, julienned

1 scallion, white and green parts, chopped

TO MAKE THE SAUCE

In a small bowl, whisk the olive oil, lemon juice, honey, and basil. Season with sea salt and set it aside.

TO MAKE THE RICE

1. In a medium saucepan over medium-high heat, combine the wild rice and enough water to cover it by 2 inches. Bring to a boil. Reduce the heat to low and simmer for about 45 minutes, or until the rice is tender. Drain the rice and transfer it to a large bowl.

2. Add the cabbage, papayas, jicama, snow peas, scallion, and sauce to the rice. Stir to mix well.

SUBSTITUTION TIP Mango, peaches, plums, and fresh pineapple could all take the place of papaya in this sweet, visually appealing meal. If the available papayas are not perfectly ripe, swap them out so the dish is sweet enough to balance the other flavors.

PER SERVING Calories: 447; Total fat: 8g; Saturated fat: 1g; Carbohydrates: 86g; Fiber: 16g; Protein: 13g

MIXED VEGETABLE STIR-FRY

SERVES 4   **PREP** 30 minutes   **COOK** 11 minutes

The usual thickeners used in stir-fries and other recipes are not allowed when you are following a rheumatoid arthritis diet because they contain gluten. Arrowroot powder is a flavorless substitution that is made from a dried root instead of grains. Arrowroot is a great source of potassium, calcium, and omega-3 fatty acids. Buying precut veggies from the produce section really helps minimize the prep too.

Vegetarian

¼ cup low-sodium vegetable broth

1 tablespoon coconut aminos

2 teaspoons raw honey

1 teaspoon grated fresh ginger

1 teaspoon bottled minced garlic

1 teaspoon arrowroot powder

1½ teaspoons sesame oil

1 cup sliced mushrooms

2 carrots, thinly sliced, or about 1 to 1½ cups precut packaged carrots

1 celery stalk, thinly sliced on an angle, or ½ cup precut packaged celery

2 cups broccoli florets

1 cup cauliflower florets

1 cup snow peas, halved

1 cup bean sprouts

¼ cup chopped cashews

1 scallion, white and green parts, chopped

1. In a small bowl, whisk the vegetable broth, coconut aminos, honey, ginger, garlic, and arrowroot powder until well combined. Set it aside.

2. In a large skillet or wok over medium-high heat, heat the sesame oil.

3. Add the mushrooms, carrots, and celery. Sauté for 4 minutes.

4. Stir in the broccoli, cauliflower, and snow peas. Sauté for about 4 minutes until crisp-tender.

5. Add the bean sprouts and sauté for 1 minute.

6. Move the vegetables to one side of the skillet and add the sauce. Cook for about 2 minutes, stirring until the sauce has thickened. Stir the vegetables into the sauce, stirring to coat.

7. Serve topped with the cashews and scallion.

SUBSTITUTION TIP Omit the cashews if you are sensitive to nuts. The sesame oil in the recipe provides enough flavor to offset their omission.

PER SERVING Calories: 154; Total fat: 6g; Saturated fat: 1g; Carbohydrates: 21g; Fiber: 4g; Protein: 7g

SESAME-QUINOA CUPS

SERVES 4 **PREP** 30 minutes

The saying, "you eat with your eyes before you eat with your mouth," is never truer than when you gaze on this stunning recipe. The deep vibrant red of the radicchio leaves and the colorful filling stand out beautifully on any plate, and the honey dressing is the perfect foil for the assertive taste.

Make Ahead

Vegetarian

FOR THE DRESSING

¼ cup olive oil

2 tablespoons rice vinegar

1 tablespoon raw honey

½ teaspoon grated
fresh ginger

½ teaspoon ground cumin

Sea salt

FOR THE CUPS

1 cup cooked quinoa

1 cup shredded carrot

1 apple, cored and chopped

1 scallion, white and green
parts, chopped

½ cup pumpkin seeds

¼ cup dried cranberries

1 tablespoon freshly
squeezed lemon juice

1 large radicchio head, core
removed, separated into
8 large leaves

1 tablespoon sesame seeds

TO MAKE THE DRESSING

In a small bowl, whisk the olive oil, rice vinegar, honey, ginger, and cumin. Season with sea salt and set it aside.

TO MAKE THE CUPS

1. In a large bowl, stir together the quinoa, carrot, apple, scallion, pumpkin seeds, cranberries, and lemon juice until well mixed.

2. Add the dressing and toss to mix well.

3. Spoon the rice mixture into the radicchio leaves, and serve topped with the sesame seeds.

VARIATION TIP Radicchio has a strong, almost astringent, taste that some people find unpleasant—despite its dazzling deep red color. Use Boston lettuce, iceberg, or romaine lettuce, with the cores removed, for a milder flavor.

PER SERVING (2 cups) Calories: 365; Total fat: 23g; Saturated fat: 4g; Carbohydrates: 34g; Fiber: 5g; Protein: 8g

THAI CABBAGE BOWL

SERVES 4 **PREP** 20 minutes **COOK** 15 minutes

Dishes described as "bowls" have popped up in some of the fanciest restaurants in the world. This designation really just means they are one-dish meals. In this recipe, the cabbage leaves serve as the bowls for the exotically spiced ingredients. You could shred the cabbage, toss it in the mix, and serve the meal in a real bowl if your cabbage leaves aren't perfect.

Make Ahead

Vegan

1 tablespoon olive oil

1 sweet onion, chopped, or about 1 cup precut packaged onion

1 teaspoon bottled minced garlic

1 teaspoon grated fresh ginger

2 cups finely chopped cauliflower

2 cups shredded broccoli stalks, or packaged broccoli slaw

1 cup shredded sweet potato

1 carrot, shredded, or ½ preshredded packaged carrots

1 cup peas (fresh or frozen and thawed)

1 cup chopped fresh spinach

2 tablespoons apple cider vinegar

1 teaspoon ground cumin

½ teaspoon ground coriander

¼ cup pumpkin seeds

¼ cup dried cherries

4 large cabbage leaves

1. Place a large skillet over medium-high heat and add the olive oil.

2. Add the onion, garlic, and ginger. Sauté for about 3 minutes, or until softened.

3. Stir in the cauliflower, broccoli, sweet potato, and carrot. Sauté for about 8 minutes, or until the vegetables are tender.

4. Stir in the peas, spinach, cider vinegar, cumin, and coriander. Sauté for about 2 minutes more until the spinach has wilted. Remove the skillet from the heat.

5. Stir in the pumpkin seeds and dried cherries. Spoon the vegetable mixture into the cabbage leaves and serve.

VARIATION TIP If you want a more substantial meal or are looking for a little more protein in your diet, add 1 cup of cooked quinoa or wild rice to the filling mixture or some meat, such as ground beef or turkey, if you want a nonvegetarian meal. If you have any filling left over, it makes a lovely side dish for another meal.

PER SERVING Calories: 208; Total fat: 8g; Saturated fat: 1g; Carbohydrates: 29g; Fiber: 8g; Protein: 8g

WILD MUSHROOM FRITTATA

SERVES 6 **PREP** 10 minutes **COOK** 40 minutes

Eggs spent at least a decade on the "naughty" list of foods because it was thought their cholesterol content contributed to heart disease. Well, it turns out cholesterol is not such a bad guy after all. It helps produce our hormones and is important for brain function. The new 2015 to 2020 USDA dietary guidelines remove the limitation on dietary cholesterol because there is no adequate evidence to recommend limiting it. Eggs do contain cholesterol, but if you are in good health it should not be a reason to avoid this nutrient-packed ingredient. They are a stellar source of protein, which can be crucial if you follow a predominantly vegetarian diet. Eggs are also very high in iron and calcium, and the yolk contains several nutrients: vitamins A, D, E, and K, and choline.

Make Ahead
Vegan

10 eggs

½ cup unsweetened almond milk

½ teaspoon ground cumin

½ teaspoon ground coriander

¼ teaspoon sea salt

1 tablespoon olive oil

2 cups sliced wild mushrooms

½ sweet onion, chopped, or about ½ cup precut packaged onion

2 teaspoons bottled minced garlic

1 tablespoon chopped fresh oregano

1. Preheat the oven to 350°F.

2. In a medium bowl, whisk the eggs, almond milk, cumin, coriander, and sea salt. Set it aside.

3. Place a large ovenproof skillet over medium-high heat and add the olive oil.

4. Add the mushrooms, onion, and garlic. Sauté for about 8 minutes, or until lightly caramelized.

5. Pour in the egg mixture and tap the skillet on the counter so the eggs flow into the vegetables.

6. Bake the frittata for about 30 minutes, or until it is cooked through and lightly browned.

7. Sprinkle with the oregano and serve.

SUBSTITUTION TIP Wild mushrooms have an incredibly diverse range of textures and flavors, but plain button or white mushrooms are delicious as well. If you can't get good-quality wild mushrooms or have a budget constraint, use the same quantity of the more common mushrooms.

PER SERVING Calories: 207; Total fat: 15g; Saturated fat: 4g; Carbohydrates: 5g; Fiber: 1g; Protein: 15g

PUMPKIN CURRY

SERVES 4   **PREP** 20 minutes   **COOK** 40 minutes

Pumpkins are probably best known for sweet pies and as festive carved decorations on Halloween. This lovely, bright ingredient is also wonderful in savory dishes even though it is actually classed as a fruit. Pumpkin contains no saturated fat and is very high in beta-carotene, vitamin A, copper, potassium, and iron. Plus, it supports healthy vision and helps cut the risk of kidney disease, cancer, and heart disease.

Make Ahead
Vegan

1 tablespoon olive oil

1 sweet onion, chopped, or about 1 cup precut packaged onion

2 teaspoons grated fresh ginger

6 cups (1-inch) pumpkin chunks

1 cup low-sodium vegetable broth

1 cup canned full-fat coconut milk

2 parsnips, diced, or 1 to 1½ cups precut packaged parsnips

1 carrot, diced, or ¾ cup precut packaged carrots

1 sweet potato, peeled and cut into 1-inch chunks, or 1½ cups precut packaged sweet potatoes

2 tablespoons Mild Curry Powder (page 50)

2 cups quartered bok choy

2 tablespoons chopped fresh cilantro

1. Place a large saucepan over medium-high heat and add the olive oil.

2. Add the onion and ginger. Sauté for about 3 minutes, or until softened.

3. Stir in the pumpkin, vegetable broth, coconut milk, parsnips, carrot, sweet potato, and curry powder. Bring the liquid to a boil. Reduce the heat to low and simmer for about 30 minutes, stirring occasionally, until the vegetables are tender and the sauce is thick and flavorful.

4. Stir in the bok choy and cook for about 5 minutes, stirring until it is tender.

5. Serve the curry topped with the cilantro.

INGREDIENT TIP Homemade vegetable stock is simple to make and the perfect way to use vegetable trimmings and extra bunches of herbs in the refrigerator. Just throw together all the carrot ends, onion peels, celery greens, and broccoli stalks in a pot of water with herbs and black peppercorns and simmer for about 2 hours. Strain and freeze the stock in sealed containers for up to 2 months.

PER SERVING Calories: 408; Total fat: 20g; Saturated fat: 14g; Carbohydrates: 59g; Fiber: 19g; Protein: 8g

WILD RICE–STUFFED SWEET POTATOES

SERVES 4 **PREP** 15 minutes **COOK** 20 minutes

Vegetables make whimsical containers for an assortment of fillings and sweet potatoes are no exception. If you have leftovers—which is unlikely—enjoy them the next day by simply reheating the stuffed sweet potato in the oven, or chop up the sweet potato's skin and flesh and mix them into the wild rice mixture. Either strategy is both simple and delicious.

Make Ahead
Vegan

2 cups cooked wild rice

½ cup shredded Swiss chard

½ cup chopped hazelnuts

½ cup dried blueberries

1 scallion, white and green parts, peeled and thinly sliced

1 teaspoon chopped fresh thyme

Sea salt

Freshly ground black pepper

4 sweet potatoes, baked in the skin until tender

1. Preheat the oven to 400°F.

2. In a medium bowl, mix together the wild rice, Swiss chard, hazelnuts, blueberries, scallion, and thyme. Season with sea salt and pepper.

3. Cut off the top third of each sweet potato, lengthwise, and scoop out most of the flesh, leaving the skin intact. Reserve the sweet potato flesh for another recipe.

4. Fill the sweet potato skins with the wild rice mixture. Place them in a 9-by-9-inch baking dish.

5. Bake the sweet potatoes for about 20 minutes, or until they are heated through. Serve warm.

SUBSTITUTION TIP Omit the hazelnuts if you react to them, and increase the wild rice by about ¼ cup. Add a finely chopped carrot to the mixture to bulk up the filling if you remove the nuts.

PER SERVING Calories: 392; Total fat: 7g; Saturated fat: 1g; Carbohydrates: 77g; Fiber: 10g; Protein: 10g

BUCKWHEAT BURGERS

SERVES 6 **PREP** 15 minutes plus 30 minutes chilling **COOK** 20 minutes

Cilantro stands up well to buckwheat and the warm spices used here, cumin and coriander. Cilantro is a superb source of calcium, iron, and vitamins A, C, and K.

Make Ahead

Vegan

1 tablespoon olive oil

1 sweet onion, chopped, or about 1 cup precut packaged onion

1 teaspoon bottled minced garlic

2 cups cooked buckwheat

1 cup almonds

¼ cup loosely packed fresh cilantro

2 tablespoons canned lite coconut milk, plus more as needed

2 teaspoons coconut aminos

1 teaspoon ground cumin

½ teaspoon ground coriander

Olive oil cooking spray

6 lettuce leaves

1. Place a medium skillet over medium-high heat and add the olive oil.

2. Add the onion and garlic. Sauté for about 4 minutes, or until lightly caramelized. Transfer to a food processor.

3. Add the buckwheat, almonds, cilantro, coconut milk, coconut aminos, cumin, and coriander to the processor. Pulse until the ingredients are finely chopped and sticking together. If the mixture is too dry and crumbly, add coconut milk by the teaspoon until the right consistency is achieved. Transfer the mixture to a bowl and divide it into 6 equal portions. Form each portion into a 3½-inch-wide burger. Refrigerate the patties for 30 minutes to firm up.

4. Preheat the broiler.

5. Place an oven rack about one-third of the distance from the top of the broiler.

6. Place the burgers on a rimmed baking sheet and spray both sides lightly with olive oil cooking spray.

7. Broil the burgers for about 7 minutes per side, until golden and heated through.

8. Serve on a lettuce leaf with your preferred toppings.

SUBSTITUTION TIP If you are sensitive to pseudo grains like buckwheat, use cooked red or green lentils instead. Substitute the same amount of lentils for the buckwheat, and adjust the liquid or add some almond flour until the burger mixture sticks together.

PER SERVING Calories: 341; Total fat: 18g; Saturated fat: 3g; Carbohydrates: 40g; Fiber: 8g; Protein: 11g

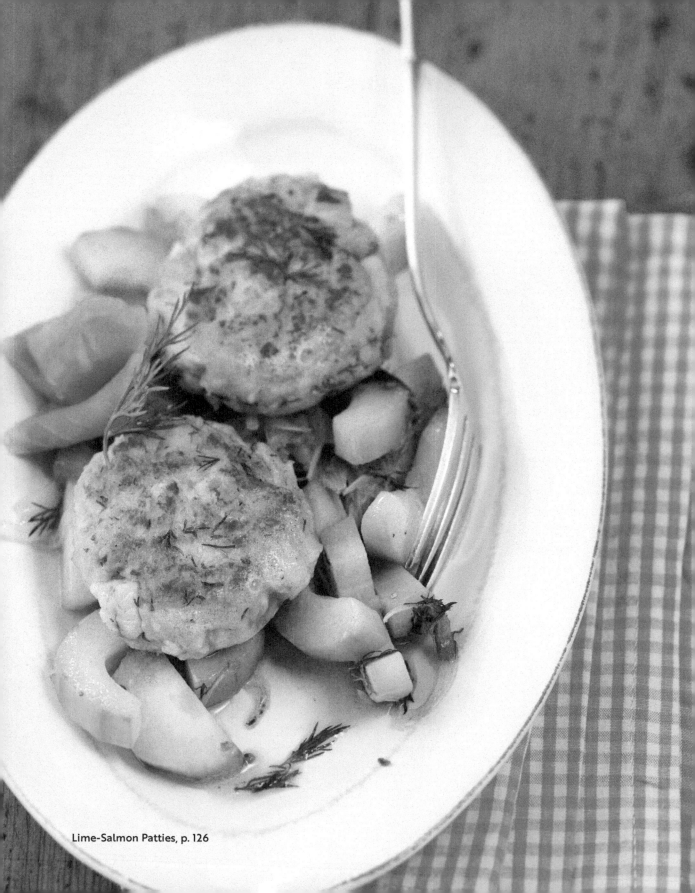

Lime-Salmon Patties, p. 126

8

FISH & SEAFOOD

MUSSELS IN HERBED BROTH

SERVES 4 **PREP** 15 minutes **COOK** 15 minutes

Choosing to eat mussels puts you in superb company because mussels have been part of meals all over the world for more than 20,000 years. They were so valued that cultivated mussel beds sprang up more than 1,000 years ago. Mussels are a tremendous source of protein—just fifteen mussels have the equivalent protein of a 6-ounce steak. This bivalve mollusk is also very high in omega-3 fatty acids and iron.

1 tablespoon olive oil

2 teaspoons bottled minced garlic

1 cup canned lite coconut milk

½ cup Herbed Chicken Bone Broth (page 76)

2 teaspoons chopped fresh thyme

1 teaspoon chopped fresh oregano

1½ pounds fresh mussels, scrubbed and debearded

1 scallion, white and green parts, thinly sliced on an angle

1. Put a large skillet over medium-high heat and add the olive oil.

2. Add the garlic. Sauté for 3 minutes, or until softened.

3. Stir in the coconut milk, chicken broth, thyme, and oregano. Bring the liquid to a boil.

4. Add the mussels. Cover the skillet and steam for about 8 minutes, or until the shells open. Discard any unopened shells and remove the skillet from the heat.

5. Stir in the scallion and serve immediately.

INGREDIENT TIP When purchasing mussels, look for closed glossy shells (or shells that close when tapped) and a fresh salty scent. Try to use the mussels the same day you purchase them; if you can't, refrigerate them covered with a cloth. Never store mussels in a sealed container, because this kills them.

PER SERVING Calories: 321; Total fat: 22g; Saturated fat: 14g; Carbohydrates: 11g; Fiber: 2g; Protein: 22g

COCONUT CRAB CAKES

SERVES 4   **PREP** 15 minutes plus 1 hour chilling   **COOK** 12 minutes

Crab is high in protein, selenium, omega-3 fatty acids, and vitamin B_{12}, while being low in calories and fat. Eating crab regularly can help protect the cardiovascular system and nervous system as well as reduce inflammation and boost the immune system.

Make Ahead

2 pounds cooked lump crabmeat, drained and picked over

½ cup shredded unsweetened coconut

½ cup coconut flour, plus more as needed

½ cup shredded carrot

2 scallions, white and green parts, finely chopped

2 eggs

1 teaspoon freshly grated lemon zest (optional)

2 tablespoons olive oil

1. In a large bowl, stir together the crab, coconut, coconut flour, carrot, scallions, eggs, and lemon zest (if using) until the mixture holds together when pressed. Add more coconut flour if the mixture is too wet.

2. Divide the mixture into 8 portions and flatten them until they are about 1 inch thick. Cover the crab cakes and refrigerate for about 1 hour to firm up.

3. Place a large skillet over medium-high heat and add the olive oil.

4. Add the crab cakes and sear for about 6 minutes per side until cooked through and golden on both sides, turning just once.

5. Serve 2 crab cakes per person.

VARIATION TIP Instead of serving these sweet crab cakes as an entrée, make delectable crab tacos for lunch. Cook them until golden, cut them in half or quarters and tuck them into lettuce leaves topped with fresh mango salsa. Delicious!

PER SERVING (2 crab cakes) Calories: 406; Total fat: 20g; Saturated fat: 8g; Carbohydrates: 5g; Fiber: 2g; Protein: 50g

LEMON ZOODLES WITH SHRIMP

SERVES 4 **PREP** 25 minutes

Shrimp is often on the favorite-food list because it is sweet, is succulent, and can be prepared successfully in many ways. Shrimp is known to be high in protein, low in fat, and low in calories as well as being a great source of selenium, vitamin B_{12}, and phosphorus. A lesser-known nutritional benefit of shrimp is the fact that it is a source of a carotenoid called astaxanthin, which can reduce the risk of cancer, boost the immune system, and support a healthy nervous system.

½ cup packed fresh basil leaves

1 teaspoon bottled minced garlic

Juice of 1 lemon (or 3 tablespoons)

Pinch sea salt

Pinch freshly ground black pepper

¼ cup canned full-fat coconut milk

1 large zucchini, julienned or spiralized

1 large yellow squash, julienned or spiralized

1 pound shrimp, deveined, boiled, peeled, and chilled

Zest of 1 lemon (optional)

1. In a food processor, combine the basil, garlic, lemon juice, sea salt, and pepper. Pulse until very finely chopped.

2. While the processor is running, add the coconut milk and blend until smooth.

3. In a large bowl, stir together the lemon-basil sauce, zucchini, and yellow squash until well coated.

4. Top the noodles with the shrimp and lemon zest (if using). Serve immediately.

VARIATION TIP This sauce is one of those versatile creations that can be made with almost any herb as a base. Try oregano, mint, dill, or even a dark leafy green like kale in the same amount as the basil.

PER SERVING Calories: 247; Total fat: 13g; Saturated fat: 5g; Carbohydrates: 5g; Fiber: 2g; Protein: 28g

SEARED SCALLOPS WITH GREENS

SERVES 4 **PREP** 20 minutes **COOK** 15 minutes

Unless you live in an area where seafood is a staple, scallops may not be in your culinary repertoire. Scallops are actually very simple to cook, and the sweet fresh taste combines well with many other ingredients. Scallops are a splendid source of protein, selenium, magnesium, and vitamin B_{12}. Use bay scallops in this recipe if they are the only product available, but they are smaller and not as sweet as sea scallops.

1½ pounds sea scallops, cleaned (see Tip) and patted dry

Sea salt

Freshly ground black pepper

2 tablespoons olive oil, divided

2 garlic cloves, thinly sliced

2 cups chopped kale leaves

2 cups fresh spinach

1. Lightly season the scallops all over with sea salt and pepper.

2. Place a large skillet over medium-high heat and add 1 tablespoon of olive oil.

3. Pan-sear the scallops for about 2 minutes per side, or until opaque and just cooked through. Transfer to a plate and cover loosely with aluminum foil to keep them warm. Wipe the skillet with a paper towel and place it back on the heat.

4. Add the remaining 1 tablespoon of olive oil to the skillet and sauté the garlic for about 4 minutes, or until caramelized.

5. Stir in the kale and spinach. Cook, tossing with tongs, for about 6 minutes, or until the greens are tender and wilted.

6. Divide the greens with any juices equally among four plates and top each with the scallops.

INGREDIENT TIP Look for slightly moist, white-fleshed scallops with smooth edges. Always buy fresh scallops because frozen ones can have a mushy texture. Make sure you remove the little rectangular-shaped side muscle from the scallops because it is tougher than the rest of the flesh.

PER SERVING Calories: 232; Total fat: 8g; Saturated fat: 1g; Carbohydrates: 9g; Fiber: 1g; Protein: 30g

PAN-SEARED HADDOCK WITH BEETS

SERVES 4 **PREP** 20 minutes **COOK** 30 minutes

Haddock is a popular choice for many dishes, including crispy battered fish and chips, because this saltwater white-fleshed fish is firm enough to handle any cooking method. Haddock is a wonderful source of protein and is high in vitamin B_3, phosphorus, and potassium. When purchasing haddock, look for fillets with translucent flesh that clings to the skin; they'll be fresh.

Make Ahead

8 beets, peeled and cut into eighths

2 shallots, thinly sliced

1 teaspoon bottled minced garlic

2 tablespoons olive oil, divided

2 tablespoons apple cider vinegar

1 teaspoon chopped fresh thyme

Pinch sea salt

4 (5-ounce) haddock fillets, patted dry

1. Preheat the oven to 400°F.

2. In a medium bowl, toss together the beets, shallots, garlic, and 1 tablespoon of olive oil until well coated. Spread the beet mixture in a 9-by-13-inch baking dish. Roast for about 30 minutes, or until the vegetables are caramelized and tender.

3. Remove the beets from the oven and stir in the cider vinegar, thyme, and sea salt.

4. While the beets are roasting, place a large skillet over medium-high heat and add the remaining 1 tablespoon of olive oil.

5. Panfry the fish for about 15 minutes, turning once, until it flakes when pressed with a fork. Serve the fish with a generous scoop of roasted beets.

INGREDIENT TIP Beets are known for their vibrant red color and rich earthy flavor. Beets also grow in other colors such as yellow, gold, white, and striped, which would be stunning in this dish. Try each variety or prepare an assortment of hues for a special guest.

PER SERVING Calories: 314; Total fat: 9g; Saturated fat: 1g; Carbohydrates: 21g; Fiber: 4g; Protein: 38g

BAKED SALMON WITH OREGANO PISTOU

SERVES 4 **PREP** 10 minutes **COOK** 20 minutes

Salmon is often the first choice for home cooks because it is a very forgiving fish with respect to cooking. Salmon is the ideal fish if you are following a healthy diet, as it is exceptionally high in omega-3 fatty acids and is a terrific source of protein, vitamin A, selenium, and calcium. It reduces inflammation in the body, supports nourished skin and hair, boosts the metabolism, and promotes a healthy cardiovascular system while cutting your risk of Alzheimer's disease.

FOR THE PISTOU

1 cup fresh oregano leaves

¼ cup almonds

2 garlic cloves

Juice of 1 lime (1 or 2 tablespoons)

Zest of 1 lime (optional)

1 tablespoon olive oil

Pinch sea salt

FOR THE FISH

4 (6-ounce) salmon fillets

Sea salt

Freshly ground black pepper

1 tablespoon olive oil

TO MAKE THE PISTOU

In a blender, combine the oregano, almonds, garlic, lime juice, lime zest (if using), olive oil, and sea salt. Pulse until very finely chopped. Transfer the pistou to a bowl and set it aside.

TO MAKE THE FISH

1. Preheat the oven to 400°F.

2. Lightly season the salmon with sea salt and pepper.

3. Place a large ovenproof skillet over medium-high heat and add the olive oil.

4. Add the salmon and pan-sear for 4 minutes per side.

5. Place the skillet in the oven and bake the fish for about 10 minutes, or until it is just cooked through.

6. Serve the salmon topped with a spoonful of pistou.

SUBSTITUTION TIP Swap out the almonds for the same amount of sunflower seeds or pumpkin seeds if you are allergic to tree nuts.

PER SERVING Calories: 377; Total fat: 22g; Saturated fat: 3g; Carbohydrates: 13g; Fiber: 9g; Protein: 36g

COCONUT MILK–BAKED SOLE

SERVES 4 **PREP** 20 minutes **COOK** 20 minutes

Using dairy products as the cooking medium is one of the best culinary methods to produce a tender flavorful protein such as fish; creamy coconut milk is an excellent substitute when dairy is not on the menu. Saffron's deep red threads infuse the coconut milk with a startling yellow color. For exceptional flavor, use the best saffron, from Spain or Iran (see Tip).

2 tablespoons warm water

Pinch saffron threads

2 pounds sole fillets

Sea salt

2 tablespoons freshly squeezed lemon juice

1 tablespoon coconut oil

1 sweet onion, chopped, or about 1 cup precut packaged onion

2 teaspoons bottled minced garlic

1 teaspoon grated fresh ginger

1 cup canned full-fat coconut milk

2 tablespoons chopped fresh cilantro

1. Place the water in a small bowl and sprinkle the saffron threads on top. Let it stand for 10 minutes.

2. Preheat the oven to 350°F.

3. Rub the fish with sea salt and the lemon juice, and place the fillets in a 9-by-9-inch baking dish. Roast the fish for 10 minutes.

4. While the fish is roasting, place a large skillet over medium-high heat and add the coconut oil.

5. Add the onion, garlic, and ginger. Sauté for about 3 minutes, or until softened.

6. Stir in the coconut milk and the saffron water. Bring to a boil. Reduce the heat to low and simmer the sauce for 5 minutes. Remove the skillet from the heat.

7. Pour the sauce over the fish. Cover and bake for about 10 minutes, or until the fish flakes easily with a fork.

8. Serve the fish topped with the cilantro.

INGREDIENT TIP Never buy ground saffron instead of threads because it can be cut with turmeric. Good-quality saffron has threads that are a uniform deep red color, are dry to the touch, and have a fragrant aroma. If you can't find saffron or it's out of your budget, substitute a pinch of turmeric. The flavor will not be the same, but the color will be similar—and the anti-inflammatory benefits remain.

PER SERVING Calories: 449; Total fat: 21g; Saturated fat: 17g; Carbohydrates: 7g; Fiber: 2g; Protein: 56g

TROUT WITH CUCUMBER SALSA

SERVES 4   **PREP** 20 minutes   **COOK** 10 minutes

Cucumber is one of those vegetables often relegated to a secondary role in salads or sandwiches, but it certainly holds its own as the base of this salsa. Cucumber is a popular detox ingredient that can reduce inflammation and the signs of aging, and lower blood pressure. This crisp, fresh vegetable is high in vitamins A, C, and K as well as potassium, magnesium, and beta-carotene.

FOR THE SALSA

1 English cucumber, diced

¼ cup unsweetened coconut yogurt

1 scallion, white and green parts, chopped

2 tablespoons chopped fresh mint

1 teaspoon raw honey

Sea salt

FOR THE FISH

1 tablespoon olive oil

4 (5-ounce) trout fillets, patted dry

Sea salt

Freshly ground black pepper

TO MAKE THE SALSA

In a small bowl, stir together the cucumber, yogurt, scallion, mint, and honey until well mixed. Season with sea salt and set it aside.

TO MAKE THE FISH

1. Place a large skillet over medium heat and add the olive oil.

2. Season the trout lightly with sea salt and pepper. Add it to the skillet and panfry for about 5 minutes per side, turning once, or until it is just cooked through.

3. Top with the cucumber salsa and serve.

SUBSTITUTION TIP Coconut yogurt can be found in most grocery stores; it has a mild, slightly nutty taste. You can also use almond yogurt or plain coconut cream (the thick layer at the top of canned coconut milk) with similar results.

PER SERVING Calories: 329; Total fat: 16g; Saturated fat: 3g; Carbohydrates: 6g; Fiber: 1g; Protein: 39g

SPICE-RUBBED SALMON WITH TANGERINE RELISH

SERVES 4 **PREP** 20 minutes **COOK** 15 minutes

Many recipes call for skinless fish fillets because the skin is often unpopular, so it makes sense to leave it off. It can be important to leave the skin on the fish, though, if you are baking it because the skin acts as a buffer between the dry heat of the oven and the moist flesh of the fillet. It also imparts flavor while keeping the fish moist. If you don't want to eat it, it can be peeled off before serving or at the table.

FOR THE RELISH

4 tangerines, peeled, segmented, and chopped

½ cup chopped jicama

1 scallion, white and green parts, chopped

2 tablespoons chopped fresh cilantro

1 teaspoon lemon zest (optional)

Pinch sea salt

FOR THE FISH

1 teaspoon ground cumin

1 teaspoon ground coriander

4 (6-ounce) skin-on salmon fillets, patted dry

1 teaspoon olive oil

TO MAKE THE RELISH

In a small bowl, stir together the tangerines, jicama, scallion, cilantro, and lemon zest (if using). Season with sea salt and set it aside.

TO MAKE THE FISH

1. Preheat the oven to 425°F.

2. In a small bowl, stir together the cumin and coriander.

3. Rub the flesh side of the fillets with the spice mixture. Arrange the salmon in a 9-by-9-inch baking dish in a single layer, skin-side up. Brush with the olive oil.

4. Bake for about 15 minutes, or until just cooked through and lightly golden.

5. Serve the fish with the salsa.

SUBSTITUTION TIP Many citrus fruits would be wonderful for this tangy salsa, such as navel oranges, Ruby Red grapefruit, or mandarin oranges. Use a combination of several types to create a colorful topping for the fish.

PER SERVING Calories: 290; Total fat: 12g; Saturated fat: 2g; Carbohydrates: 14g; Fiber: 2g; Protein: 34g

BAKED HALIBUT WITH AVOCADO SALSA

SERVES 4 **PREP** 20 minutes **COOK** 15 minutes

Mangos add sweetness and color to the tasty salsa topping this dish. This gorgeous fruit is the epitome of exotic with its luscious silky texture and vibrant yellow flesh. Mangos can be tricky to cut because their pit is rectangular instead of round or oval, so don't get frustrated if you have difficulties. Use the leftover mango in this recipe for a smoothie, as a salad topping, or as a delicious healthy snack.

FOR THE SALSA

1 avocado, peeled, pitted, and diced

½ mango, diced, or about 1 cup frozen chunks, thawed

½ cup chopped fresh strawberries

1 teaspoon chopped fresh mint

Juice of 1 lemon (3 tablespoons)

Zest of 1 lemon (optional)

FOR THE FISH

4 (6-ounce) boneless skinless halibut fillets, patted dry

Sea salt

Freshly ground black pepper

1 tablespoon olive oil

TO MAKE THE SALSA

In a medium bowl, stir together the avocado, mango, strawberries, mint, lemon juice, and lemon zest (if using). Set it aside.

TO MAKE THE FISH

1. Lightly season the halibut with sea salt and pepper.

2. Place a large skillet over medium heat and add the olive oil.

3. Add the fish and panfry for about 7 minutes per side, turning once, or until it is just cooked through.

4. Top with the avocado salsa and serve.

VARIATION TIP The strawberries in the salsa are meant to add a vibrant splash of color for visual appeal. You can use other brightly hued fruits or vegetables for the same effect. Try radish, watermelon, red cabbage, red onion, Ruby Red grapefruit, or even pomegranate arils.

PER SERVING Calories: 354; Total fat: 15g; Saturated fat: 3g; Carbohydrates: 12g; Fiber: 4g; Protein: 43g

LIME-SALMON PATTIES

SERVES 4 **PREP** 20 minutes plus 30 minutes chilling **COOK** 10 minutes

These citrus-infused fish cakes are delightful served alone with a lime wedge and a nice quinoa side dish, but they can also be served—either warm or cold—on top of a fresh cucumber salad. As with most burgers, the patties freeze easily with a piece of parchment paper between each and tucked in a sealable freezer bag. Simply take out what you need and thaw them in the refrigerator overnight. Rewarm in a low (200°F) oven for about 6 minutes, turning at least once.

Make Ahead

½ pound cooked boneless salmon fillet, flaked

2 eggs

¾ cup almond flour, plus more as needed

1 scallion, white and green parts, chopped

Juice of 2 limes (2 to 4 tablespoons), plus more as needed

Zest of 2 limes (optional)

1 tablespoon chopped fresh dill

Pinch sea salt

1 tablespoon olive oil

1 lime, cut into wedges

1. In a large bowl, mix together the salmon, eggs, almond flour, scallion, lime juice, lime zest (if using), dill, and sea salt until the mixture holds together when pressed. If the mixture is too dry, add more lime juice; if it is too wet, add more almond flour.

2. Divide the salmon mixture into 4 equal portions, and press them into patties about ½ inch thick. Refrigerate them for about 30 minutes to firm up.

3. Place a large skillet over medium-high heat and add the olive oil.

4. Add the salmon patties and brown for about 5 minutes per side, turning once.

5. Serve the patties with lime wedges.

SUBSTITUTION TIP This recipe calls for cooked salmon with the assumption you will cook a raw piece of fish or use leftovers from another meal. You can use good-quality water-packed canned salmon if you want to save time and money.

PER SERVING Calories: 243; Total fat: 18g; Saturated fat: 2g; Carbohydrates: 5g; Fiber: 2g; Protein: 18g

FISH AND VEGETABLE CASSEROLE

SERVES 4 **PREP** 25 minutes **COOK** 30 minutes

Parsnip joins other sweet root vegetables in this convenient and appealing casserole. Although it might look like a pale version of a carrot, the humble parsnip has a unique taste all its own. You probably would not describe it as sweet until roasting it, which brings out its natural sugars. Parsnips are very high in fiber and potassium while being low in calories. Eating them can help regulate blood sugar and cut the risk of developing cardiovascular disease and dementia. Using precut vegetables purchased from the produce section can help with prep here.

Make Ahead

2 cups diced sweet potato

2 cups diced carrot

2 cups diced parsnip

1 sweet onion, cut into eighths

1 cup (2-inch) asparagus pieces

2 teaspoons chopped fresh thyme

1 teaspoon bottled minced garlic

¼ teaspoon sea salt

1 tablespoon olive oil

4 (6-ounce) skinless tilapia fillets

Juice of 1 lemon (3 tablespoons)

1. Preheat the oven to 350°F.

2. Tear off four 18-by-24-inch pieces of aluminum foil and fold each piece in half to make four 18-by-12-inch pieces.

3. In a large bowl, toss together the sweet potato, carrot, parsnip, onion, asparagus, thyme, garlic, sea salt, and olive oil. Place one-fourth of the vegetables in the center of each foil piece.

4. Top each vegetable mound with one tilapia fillet.

5. Sprinkle the fish with lemon juice.

6. Fold the foil to create sealed packages that have a bit of space at the top, and arrange the packets on a baking sheet.

7. Bake for about 30 minutes, or until the fish begins to flake and the vegetables are tender.

8. Carefully open the packets, plate, and serve.

COOKING TIP The cooking technique used for this dish is meant to steam the fish and vegetables to form a tender, flavorful finished dish. Instead of individual packages, use a traditional casserole dish and bake it, covered, to produce a similar effect.

PER SERVING Calories: 353; Total fat: 6g; Saturated fat: 1g; Carbohydrates: 43g; Fiber: 9g; Protein: 36g

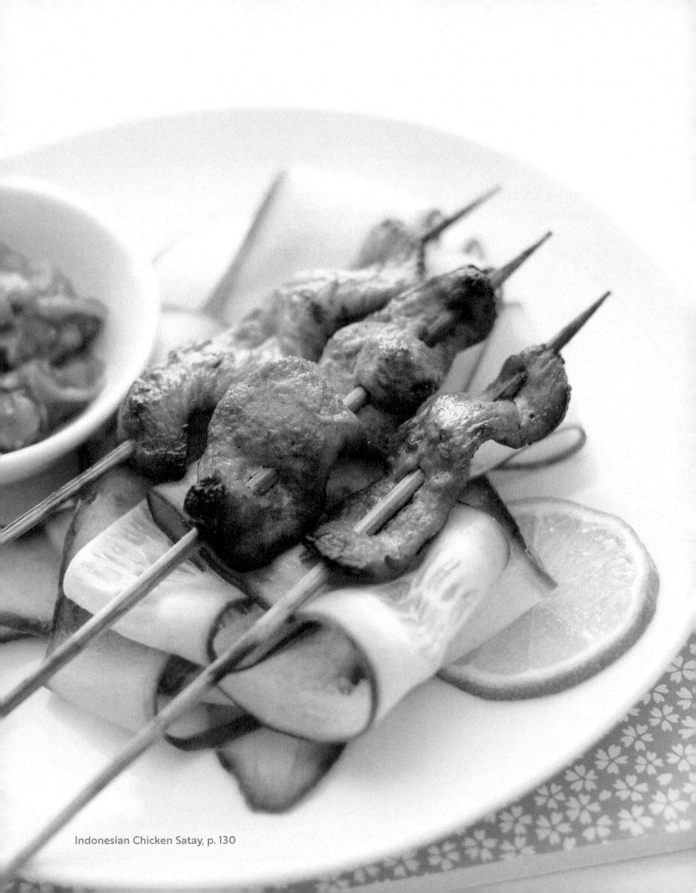

Indonesian Chicken Satay, p. 130

9

POULTRY & MEAT

INDONESIAN CHICKEN SATAY

SERVES 4 **PREP** 15 minutes plus 1 hour to marinate **COOK** 8 minutes

The traditional Indonesian satay sauce has a generous pinch of red pepper flakes to provide heat; however, red pepper flakes are a nightshade spice, so they cannot be consumed on a rheumatoid arthritis diet. Fresh ginger adds the heat here instead, along with lots of flavor and health benefits. Ginger is a known remedy for digestive problems as well as a potent anti-inflammatory that can help relieve the symptoms of arthritis.

FOR THE SAUCE

½ cup almond butter

¼ cup water

2 tablespoons coconut aminos

1 tablespoon grated fresh ginger

1 tablespoon freshly squeezed lime juice

1 garlic clove

1 teaspoon raw honey

FOR THE SATAY

Juice of 2 limes (2 to 4 tablespoons)

2 tablespoons olive oil

2 tablespoons raw honey

1 tablespoon finely chopped fresh cilantro

1 tablespoon bottled minced garlic

1½ pounds boneless skinless chicken breast, cut into strips

TO MAKE THE SAUCE

In a blender, combine the almond butter, water, coconut aminos, ginger, lime juice, garlic, and honey. Pulse until smooth. Set it aside.

TO MAKE THE SATAY

1. In a large bowl, whisk the lime juice, olive oil, honey, cilantro, and garlic until well mixed.

2. Add the chicken strips and toss to coat. Cover the bowl with plastic wrap and refrigerate for 1 hour to marinate.

3. Preheat the broiler.

4. Place a rack in the upper quarter of the oven.

5. Thread each chicken strip onto a wooden skewer, and lay them on a rimmed baking sheet.

6. Broil the chicken for about 4 minutes per side until cooked through and golden, turning once.

7. Serve with the sauce.

VARIATION TIP Traditional Indonesian satay uses a spicy peanut sauce, so my almond butter version is not traditional. Omit the sauce completely if tree nuts are an allergen in your household.

PER SERVING Calories: 181; Total fat: 11g; Saturated fat: 2g; Carbohydrates: 12g; Fiber: 0g; Protein: 10g

HERB-ROASTED CHICKEN

SERVES 4   **PREP** 15 minutes   **COOK** 1 hour, 30 minutes

The tantalizing aroma of roasting chicken with hints of citrus and herbs will fill your entire house. Getting your family to the dinner table will never be easier. Leftover roast chicken is wonderful because you can use all the parts. Save the carcass for Herbed Chicken Bone Broth (page 76), and the meat for other recipes such as salads, soups, and casseroles.

1 (4-pound) whole chicken, rinsed and patted dry

2 lemons, halved

1 sweet onion, quartered

4 garlic cloves, crushed

6 fresh thyme sprigs

6 fresh rosemary sprigs

3 bay leaves

2 tablespoons olive oil

Sea salt

Freshly ground black pepper

1. Preheat the oven to 400°F.

2. Place the chicken in a roasting pan. Stuff the lemons, onion, garlic, thyme, rosemary, and bay leaves into the cavity. Brush the chicken with the olive oil, and season lightly with sea salt and pepper.

3. Roast the chicken for about 1½ hours until golden brown and cooked through.

4. Remove the chicken from the oven and let it sit for 10 minutes. Remove the lemons, onion, and herbs from the cavity and serve.

VARIATION TIP Instead of stuffing the herbs into the cavity of the chicken, gently lift the skin of the breast and tuck the herbs and a little citrus zest between the skin and breast meat. Roast and carve the bird as you usually would, with the herbs still in place.

PER SERVING Calories: 261; Total fat: 9g; Saturated fat: 2g; Carbohydrates: 5g; Fiber: 2g; Protein: 38g

COCONUT-BRAISED CHICKEN

SERVES 4 **PREP** 15 minutes **COOK** 35 minutes

This sweet citrus-and-ginger sauce is delightful spooned over golden chicken thighs and topped with bright green scallions. Thighs have more flavor than the breasts, and the added skin does not add too many calories or fat grams to the finished dish. If you want to create a dish that supports weight-loss goals, remove the skin either before or after the chicken is cooked.

1½ cups canned lite coconut milk

2 tablespoons grated fresh ginger

Juice of 1 lime (1 or 2 tablespoons)

Zest of 1 lime (optional)

1 tablespoon raw honey

½ teaspoon ground cardamom

1 tablespoon olive oil

1 pound bone-in skin-on chicken thighs

1 scallion, white and green parts, chopped

1. In a medium bowl, whisk the coconut milk, ginger, lime juice, lime zest (if using), honey, and cardamom. Set it aside.

2. Place a large skillet over medium-high heat and add the olive oil.

3. Add the chicken thighs and pan-sear for about 20 minutes, or until golden, turning once.

4. Pour the coconut milk mixture over the chicken, and bring the liquid to a boil. Reduce the heat to low, cover, and simmer for about 15 minutes, or until the chicken is tender and cooked through.

5. Serve garnished with the scallions.

VARIATION TIP Chicken thighs are often overlooked, which is unfortunate because they are juicy and flavorful. If chicken breasts are your preferred cut of poultry, swap out the thighs and cook the breasts in the same manner.

PER SERVING Calories: 480; Total fat: 34g; Saturated fat: 22g; Carbohydrates: 12g; Fiber: 3g; Protein: 35g

CHICKEN BUCKWHEAT FLORENTINE

SERVES 6 **PREP** 20 minutes **COOK** 45 minutes

"Florentine" means "in the manner of Florence" and in cooking it means the use of spinach. Catherine de Médicis, a sixteenth-century French queen from Florence, Italy, introduced spinach to the French court and even brought spinach seeds with her to France. Spinach is one of the most nutritious foods in the world: it contains almost 1,000 percent of the daily recommended amount (RDA) of vitamin K and 100 percent of the RDA of vitamin A.

Make Ahead

1 tablespoon olive oil

3 (8-ounce) boneless skinless chicken breasts, diced

1 sweet onion, chopped, or about 1 cup precut packaged onion

2 cups sliced button mushrooms

2 teaspoons bottled minced garlic

1 cup uncooked buckwheat

1 cup Herbed Chicken Bone Broth (page 76)

1 cup canned lite coconut milk

½ teaspoon ground nutmeg

4 cups fresh spinach

Sea salt

Zest of 1 lemon (optional)

1. Place a skillet over medium-high heat and add the olive oil.

2. Add the chicken. Sauté for about 15 minutes, turning once, until just cooked through. With a slotted spoon, remove the chicken to a plate and set it aside. Return the skillet to the heat.

3. Add the onion, mushrooms, and garlic to the skillet. Sauté for about 5 minutes, or until softened.

4. Pour in the buckwheat and sauté for 1 minute.

5. Stir in the chicken broth, coconut milk, and nutmeg. Bring the liquid to a boil. Reduce the heat to low and simmer, covered, for about 25 minutes, or until the buckwheat is tender.

6. Stir in the spinach and chicken, and season with sea salt.

7. Serve sprinkled with lemon zest (if using).

SUBSTITUTION TIP Buckwheat is a mainstay of Russian and Eastern Europe cuisines. If you aren't a fan of its earthy flavor, use the same quantity of quinoa.

PER SERVING Calories: 490; Total fat: 22g; Saturated fat: 11g; Carbohydrates: 37g; Fiber: 6g; Protein: 40g

TURKEY-THYME MEATBALLS

SERVES 4 **PREP** 20 minutes **COOK** 15 minutes

Turkey is often combined with different herbs, especially when roasted, but the earthy, almost licorice-like flavor of thyme meshes perfectly with it. Thyme is a superb source of vitamins A and C as well as iron and copper. Herbs such as thyme are also considered to be powerful medicinal tools and have been used for centuries to reduce the symptoms of ailments and provide relief. Thyme was often used to treat cough and congestion, especially in the winter.

Make Ahead

1½ pounds lean ground turkey

½ sweet onion, chopped, or about ½ cup precut packaged onion

¼ cup almond flour

1 tablespoon chopped fresh thyme

2 teaspoons bottled minced garlic

1 egg

¼ teaspoon ground nutmeg

Pinch sea salt

1. Preheat the oven to 350°F.

2. Line a rimmed baking sheet with aluminum foil and set it aside.

3. In a large bowl, combine the turkey, onion, almond flour, thyme, garlic, egg, nutmeg, and sea salt until well mixed. Roll the turkey mixture into 1½-inch meatballs. Arrange the meatballs on the prepared baking sheet.

4. Bake for about 15 minutes, or until browned and cooked through.

SUBSTITUTION TIP The egg could be left out of the mixture to avoid allergens, but if you do so, add 2 tablespoons of unsweetened almond milk to keep the liquid ratio.

PER SERVING Calories: 303; Total fat: 16g; Saturated fat: 4g; Carbohydrates: 4g; Fiber: 1g; Protein: 36g

PORK TENDERLOIN WITH SAVORY BERRY SAUCE

SERVES 4 **PREP** 20 minutes **COOK** 20 minutes plus 10 minutes resting

Fruit sauces and roasted meat are a perfect marriage of savory and sweet and are particularly popular in colder months. Blueberries are an exceptional choice because they are available year-round and are a superfood. Superfoods can fight degenerative diseases, boost your immune system, and help lower blood pressure. Blueberries are packed with antioxidants, phytonutrients, folic acid, vitamin B_1, potassium, and calcium.

FOR THE PORK

2 (10-ounce) pork tenderloins, trimmed and patted dry

Sea salt

Freshly ground black pepper

1 tablespoon olive oil

TO MAKE THE PORK

1. Preheat the oven to 425°F.

2. Lightly season the tenderloins with sea salt and pepper.

3. Place a medium ovenproof skillet over medium-high heat and add the olive oil.

4. Add the pork. Brown it on all sides, turning, for about 5 minutes total.

5. Place the skillet in the oven and roast the pork for about 15 minutes until just cooked through. Remove from the oven and let the pork rest for 10 minutes.

6. Slice the pork into medallions and serve with the berry sauce.

FOR THE SAUCE

1 tablespoon olive oil

¼ cup finely chopped sweet onion

½ cup Herbed Chicken Bone Broth (page 76)

2 tablespoons apple cider vinegar

1 cup fresh blueberries

¼ teaspoon ground nutmeg

1 teaspoon lemon zest (optional)

TO MAKE THE SAUCE

1. While the pork roasts, place a small saucepan over medium-high heat and add the olive oil.

2. Add the onion. Sauté for about 3 minutes, or until softened.

3. Stir in the chicken broth and cider vinegar. Bring the liquid to a boil. Reduce the heat to low and simmer for about 4 minutes, or until the sauce has reduced by half.

4. Stir in the blueberries and nutmeg. Cook for about 5 minutes, or until the berries break down. Remove the sauce from the heat and stir in the lemon zest (if using).

5. Serve with the pork medallions.

INGREDIENT TIP Pork tenderloin sometimes needs to be cleaned before cooking to remove the thin silverskin. Insert a thin, sharp boning knife tip under this shiny connective tissue, and cut it off without removing too much flesh. The reason for removing it is that silverskin will not dissolve when the pork is cooked.

PER SERVING Calories: 375; Total fat: 19g; Saturated fat: 5g; Carbohydrates: 6g; Fiber: 1g; Protein: 43g

PORK CHOPS WITH COOKED APPLE SALSA

SERVES 4 **PREP** 20 minutes **COOK** 25 minutes

Pork has come a long way in terms of how it is cooked and what internal temperature is considered safe. Pork used to be cooked to the point of dryness to avoid contracting a parasite called trichinae, which lived in pork meat. Trichinae is not really a concern anymore and the U.S. Department of Agriculture now states that cooking pork to an internal temperature of 145°F is perfectly acceptable, so your chops will have a hint of juicy pink through the center.

FOR THE SALSA

1 teaspoon olive oil

¼ cup finely chopped sweet onion

½ teaspoon grated fresh ginger

2 apples, peeled, cored, and diced

½ cup dried raisins

Pinch sea salt

FOR THE PORK CHOPS

4 (4-ounce) boneless center-cut pork chops, trimmed and patted dry

1 teaspoon garlic powder

1 teaspoon ground cinnamon

Sea salt

Freshly ground black pepper

1 tablespoon olive oil

TO MAKE THE SALSA

1. Place a medium skillet over medium heat and add the olive oil.

2. Add the onion and ginger. Sauté for about 2 minutes, or until softened.

3. Stir in the apples and raisins. Sauté for about 5 minutes, or until the fruit is just tender. Season the salsa with sea salt and set it aside.

TO MAKE THE PORK CHOPS

1. Sprinkle the pork chops on both sides with the garlic powder, cinnamon, sea salt, and pepper.

2. Place a large skillet over medium-high heat and add the olive oil.

3. Add the seasoned chops and panfry for 7 to 8 minutes per side until just cooked through and browned, turning once.

4. Serve the chops with the cooked apple salsa.

VARIATION TIP Sweet potatoes make for a filling and vitamin-rich addition to this meal. If you have time, prepare in advance Slow-Roasted Sweet Potatoes (page 67). After roasting, mash them well with a fork or add to the food processor and pulse until you get a slightly chunky mash, as pictured on page 2.

PER SERVING Calories: 434; Total fat: 32g; Saturated fat: 11g; Carbohydrates: 10g; Fiber: 1g; Protein: 26g

PORK LOIN WITH ROASTED FENNEL AND CELERIAC

SERVES 4   **PREP** 15 minutes   **COOK** 1 hour, 15 minutes plus 10 minutes resting

Roasting fennel creates a luscious mellow flavor with a strong licorice undertone that blends beautifully with the fresh celery taste of the celeriac. Fennel is an elegant vegetable whose feathery fronds are perfect for a garnish or tossed into a smoothie the next day. Fennel is very high in B vitamins, vitamin C, potassium, and iron, which all support a healthy cardiovascular system. Use a food processor to prep the fennel and celeriac if the chopping is too difficult for you.

1 fennel bulb, fronds cut off, cut into ¼-inch slices

1 celeriac, peeled and diced

2 tablespoons olive oil, divided

1 tablespoon pure maple syrup

1 teaspoon bottled minced garlic

Pinch sea salt

1 pound boned pork loin, trimmed of visible fat

1 teaspoon chopped fresh thyme

1. Preheat the oven to 375°F.

2. In a large bowl, toss the fennel, celeriac, 1 tablespoon of olive oil, maple syrup, garlic, and sea salt until well mixed. Transfer the vegetables to a 9-by-13-inch baking dish and set it aside.

3. Place a large skillet over medium-high heat, and add the remaining 1 tablespoon of olive oil.

4. Add the pork loin. Brown it on all sides, turning, for about 15 minutes total. Place the browned pork on top on the vegetables and sprinkle with the thyme.

5. Roast the pork for about 1 hour until cooked through but still juicy.

6. Transfer the roast and vegetables to a serving platter and pour any pan juices over the top.

7. Let the meat rest for 10 minutes before serving.

VARIATION TIP Other delicious choices to pair with fennel in this dish are apples, pears, parsnip, sweet potato, and turnip. Substitute about 3 cups of your alternative choice for the celeriac, and keep all other ingredients the same.

PER SERVING Calories: 400; Total fat: 23g; Saturated fat: 7g; Carbohydrates: 15g; Fiber: 3g; Protein: 33g

GRAINY MUSTARD–CRUSTED LAMB

SERVES 4 **PREP** 10 minutes **COOK** 35 minutes plus 10 minutes resting

Lamb and rosemary are often paired together because this herb has an assertive flavor that is not lost in the gamey taste of the meat. Rosemary stems are hard and woody so, unlike many other herbs, it is best to strip the leaves from the stems before chopping. This pungent herb can help detoxify the liver and fight inflammation due to its high levels of vitamins A and C as well as calcium and iron.

¼ cup whole-grain Dijon mustard

2 tablespoons chopped fresh thyme

1 tablespoon chopped fresh rosemary

2 (8-rib) frenched lamb racks, patted dry

Sea salt

Freshly ground black pepper

1 tablespoon olive oil

1. Preheat the oven to 425°F.

2. In a small bowl, stir together the mustard, thyme, and rosemary.

3. Lightly season the lamb racks with sea salt and pepper.

4. Place a large ovenproof skillet over medium-high heat and add the olive oil.

5. Add the lamb racks. Pan-sear for about 2 minutes per side, turning once. Remove the skillet from the heat.

6. Turn the racks upright in the skillet with the bones interlaced, and spread the mustard mixture over the outside surface of the lamb. Roast for about 30 minutes for medium, or until your desired doneness.

7. Remove the lamb racks from the oven and let them rest for 10 minutes. Cut the racks into chops and serve 4 per person.

INGREDIENT TIP Arrange with your butcher to french the lamb racks before you take them home, or purchase them already prepared in this manner. Frenching means to remove the excess fat and connective tissue from the rib bone, and can be a time-consuming task, especially if you do not own a sharp boning knife.

PER SERVING (4 chops) Calories: 469; Total fat: 21g; Saturated fat: 7g; Carbohydrates: 2g; Fiber: 1g; Protein: 65g

LAMB SOUVLAKI

MAKES 8 skewers   **PREP** 10 minutes plus 1 hour marinating   **COOK** 15 minutes

Lamb used to be imported meat that was expensive and hard to obtain. It is now farmed throughout North America, and farming techniques are producing leaner animals that have less saturated fat. About 50 percent of the fat found on these animals is monounsaturated. Lamb is also a fabulous source of B vitamins, iron, and zinc.

2 tablespoons olive oil

2 tablespoons apple cider vinegar

1 tablespoon dried oregano

2 teaspoons bottled minced garlic

½ teaspoon sea salt

1 pound lamb shoulder, cut into 1-inch cubes

1. In a large bowl, stir together the olive oil, cider vinegar, oregano, garlic, and sea salt until well mixed.

2. Stir in the lamb. Cover the bowl and refrigerate it for 1 hour to marinate.

3. Preheat the broiler.

4. Place one of the racks in the upper third of the oven.

5. Using 8 wooden skewers, thread 4 or 5 pieces of lamb on each and arrange them on a baking sheet.

6. Broil, turning, for about 15 minutes total until the meat is browned evenly on all sides.

COOKING TIP If you own a barbeque, these tender kebabs are wonderful grilled. If you are grilling the lamb, soak the wooden skewers for 30 minutes in water before threading on the meat so they do not char to pieces over the heat.

PER SERVING (2 skewers) Calories: 278; Total fat: 15g; Saturated fat: 4g; Carbohydrates: 1g; Fiber: 1g; Protein: 32g

MOROCCAN LAMB STEW

SERVES 4 **PREP** 25 minutes **COOK** 2 hours, 15 minutes

The beauty of a good stew is that it comes together easily after the initial prep work. This stew can be simmered on the stove top, braised in the oven, or made in a convenient slow cooker so it is ready when you walk in the door after a long day. Serve the stew over cauliflower rice or fluffy quinoa for a filling meal.

Make Ahead

2 tablespoons olive oil, divided

1 pound lamb shoulder, trimmed of visible fat and cut into 1-inch chunks

2 stalks celery, chopped, or about ¾ to 1 cup precut packaged celery

1 sweet onion, chopped, or about 1 cup precut packaged onion

1 tablespoon grated fresh ginger

2 teaspoons bottled minced garlic

1 teaspoon ground cinnamon

½ teaspoon ground turmeric

¼ teaspoon ground allspice

2 cups Beef Bone Broth (page 78)

2 cups diced sweet potato

1 cup diced carrot

1 cup diced parsnip

2 cups fresh spinach

2 tablespoons chopped fresh parsley

1. Preheat the oven to 325°F.

2. Place a large ovenproof skillet over medium-high heat and add 1 tablespoon of olive oil.

3. Add the lamb in batches. Brown for about 8 minutes total. With a slotted spoon, remove the meat to a plate. Return the skillet to the heat.

4. To the skillet, add the remaining 1 tablespoon of olive oil, the celery, onion, ginger, and garlic. Sauté for about 3 minutes, or until softened.

5. Stir in the cinnamon, turmeric, and allspice. Sauté for 1 minute.

6. Stir in the beef broth, lamb, and any accumulated juices on the plate, the sweet potato, carrot, and parsnip. Bring the liquid to a boil. Cover the skillet and place it in the oven. Braise the stew for about 2 hours, stirring occasionally, until the lamb is very tender.

7. Remove the stew from the oven and stir in the spinach.

8. Let the stew sit for 10 minutes. Serve garnished with the parsley.

INGREDIENT TIP Lamb shoulder is a lovely cut to make into stew if you trim off the fat completely before browning it. Lamb leg, shanks, and neck are also great choices for slow cooking.

PER SERVING Calories: 432; Total fat: 16g; Saturated fat: 4g; Carbohydrates: 35g; Fiber: 7g; Protein: 37g

BEEF SIRLOIN KEBABS IN GARLIC MARINADE

SERVES 4 **PREP** 20 minutes plus 1 hour to marinating **COOK** 10 minutes plus 5 minutes resting

The delectable taste of garlic enriches every bite of this simple dish. Garlic contains more than 70 phytonutrients and a broad range of other nutrients such as vitamin B_1, calcium, fiber, manganese, and selenium. Eating garlic regularly can help fight the common cold, reduce the risk of cancer, and promote a healthy cardiovascular system. If you are buying fresh garlic in bulbs, look for a heavy, firm bulb with no soft spots.

2 tablespoons olive oil, divided

1 tablespoon coconut aminos

1 tablespoon apple cider vinegar

1 tablespoon bottled minced garlic

1 tablespoon chopped fresh cilantro

1 pound boneless top sirloin steak, trimmed of visible fat and cut into 1½-inch chunks

1 red onion, quartered and separated into layers

1 sweet potato, peeled, halved lengthwise, and each half cut into 8 pieces

8 medium button mushrooms

1. In a large bowl, stir together 1 tablespoon of olive oil, the coconut aminos, cider vinegar, garlic, and cilantro until well mixed.

2. Add the beef to the bowl and stir to coat the meat in the marinade. Cover the bowl and refrigerate for 1 hour to marinate.

3. Preheat the broiler.

4. Place an oven rack in the top quarter of the oven.

5. On 4 skewers, assemble the kebabs by alternating pieces of beef, onion, sweet potato, and mushrooms.

6. Lightly brush the vegetables with the remaining 1 tablespoon of olive oil, and arrange the kebabs on a baking sheet.

7. Broil the kebabs for 10 minutes for medium, turning once or twice, or until the beef is cooked to your desired doneness. Transfer the kebabs to a plate, and let them rest for 5 minutes before serving.

SUBSTITUTION TIP One of the best parts of making kebabs is that you can thread almost anything on the skewers and get a lovely meal. If you are short of any of the vegetable choices in the recipe, double up on the others or make straight beef kebabs.

PER SERVING (1 kebab) Calories: 319; Total fat: 14g; Saturated fat: 4g; Carbohydrates: 10g; Fiber: 2g; Protein: 37g

SAVORY BEEF MEATLOAF

SERVES 4 **PREP** 10 minutes **COOK** 1 hour plus 10 minutes resting

Meatloaf is one of the easiest recipes to make, so it is not surprising that many home cooks and chefs try to complicate the recipe with exotic ingredients and unnecessary cooking techniques. This is a simple recipe featuring lean beef, onion, herbs, and a little fresh horseradish for a satisfying kick. Although regular ground beef has more flavor, it produces a meatloaf that requires the purged grease to be tipped out of the loaf pan, so stick to extra lean.

Make Ahead

1½ pounds extra-lean ground beef

½ cup almond flour

½ cup chopped sweet onion

1 egg

1 tablespoon chopped fresh basil

1 tablespoon chopped fresh parsley

1 teaspoon grated fresh horseradish, or prepared horseradish

⅛ teaspoon sea salt

1. Preheat the oven to 350°F.

2. In a large bowl, combine the ground beef, almond flour, onion, egg, basil, parsley, horseradish, and sea salt until well mixed. Press the meatloaf mixture into a 9-by-5-inch loaf pan.

3. Bake for about 1 hour until cooked through.

4. Remove the meatloaf from the oven, and let it rest for 10 minutes.

SUBSTITUTION TIP Egg in meatloaf is usually a binder, but it can be left out if you have an allergy. Increase the almond flour by 2 tablespoons if egg is an issue.

PER SERVING Calories: 407; Total fat: 18g; Saturated fat: 5g; Carbohydrates: 4g; Fiber: 2g; Protein: 56g

BUCKWHEAT CABBAGE ROLLS

SERVES 4 **PREP** 30 minutes **COOK** 1 hour, 5 minutes

Cabbage rolls use only about 10 percent of the cabbage head because you peel off the largest outer leaves to use as wrappers. Leftover cabbage can be turned into lovely creamy coleslaw or fermented into tangy healthy sauerkraut if you have a little time to sterilize jars. Sauerkraut is a probiotic food that can help heal the gut and is an important part of any diet addressing autoimmune diseases.

8 large outer cabbage leaves with the hard core removed

1 pound lean ground beef

½ cup cooked buckwheat

½ sweet onion, chopped, or about ½ cup precut packaged onion

1 egg

2 teaspoons bottled minced garlic

1 teaspoon chopped fresh oregano

Pinch sea salt

½ cup Beef Bone Broth (page 78)

1. Preheat the oven to 350°F.

2. Fill a large saucepan with water, place it over high heat, and bring to a boil.

3. Add the cabbage leaves. Blanch for about 4 minutes, or until tender. Remove them from the water and set them aside.

4. In a large bowl, combine the ground beef, buckwheat, onion, egg, garlic, oregano, and sea salt until well mixed. Divide the mixture into 8 portions.

5. Place 1 cabbage leaf on a work surface, and place 1 meat portion in the center. Fold the sides of the leaf over the meat. Roll the leaf from the nearest unfolded edge until the meat is completely enclosed in a roll. Place the roll seam-side down in a 9-by-9-inch baking dish. Repeat with the remaining leaves and meat portions.

6. Pour the beef broth over the cabbage rolls. Cover the baking dish with aluminum foil, and bake for about 1 hour until the filling is cooked through.

SUBSTITUTION TIP The traditional sauce for cabbage rolls contains tomatoes, which are a member of the nightshade family and not recommended on this diet. If you want a thicker sauce, double the beef broth in the recipe, remove the rolls when they are cooked, and thicken the broth with a little arrowroot powder.

PER SERVING Calories: 380; Total fat: 8g; Saturated fat: 3g; Carbohydrates: 35g; Fiber: 5g; Protein: 41g

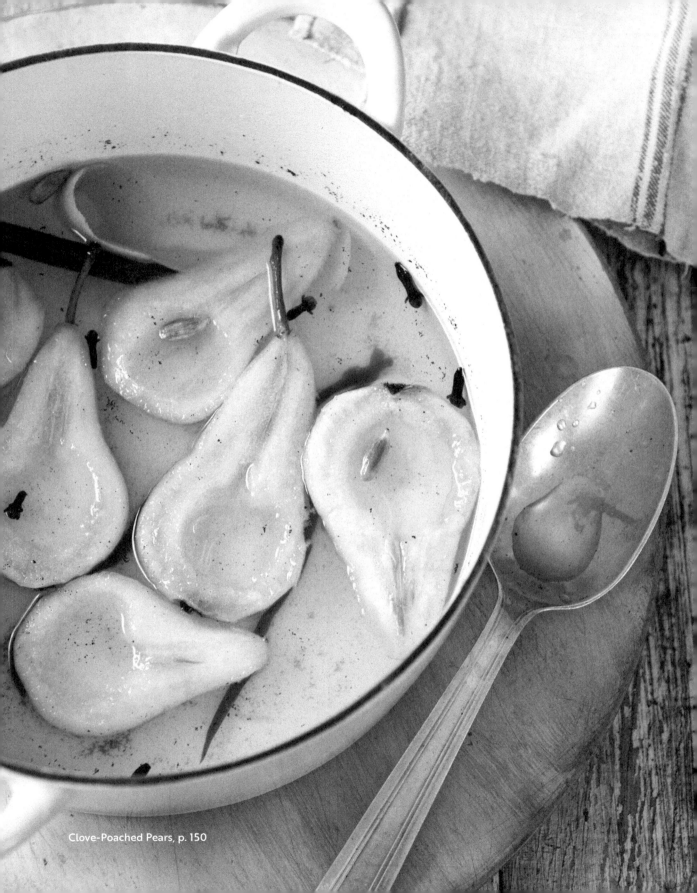

Clove-Poached Pears, p. 150

10

DESSERTS

ALMOND-QUINOA CRISPS

SERVES 8 **PREP** 10 minutes plus 1 hour chilling

If you need an unassuming dessert to serve after a casual picnic or a less-filling choice after a large meal, look no further than these crispy bars. Puffed quinoa can be found in the organic section of your supermarket or in a health food store. You are probably familiar with puffed rice snacks packed with sugar and fat, so this healthy version will come as a delightful guilt-free treat.

Make Ahead

Vegetarian

Coconut oil, for greasing the baking dish

½ cup almond butter

¼ cup raw honey

¼ cup carob powder

4 cups puffed quinoa

¼ cup chopped almonds

1. Lightly grease an 8-by-8-inch baking dish with coconut oil and set it aside.

2. In a small saucepan over low heat, add the almond butter, honey, and carob powder, and stir until the ingredients are thoroughly mixed, smooth, and melted. Remove the saucepan from the heat.

3. In a large bowl, toss together the quinoa and almonds.

4. Add the almond butter mixture. Stir everything together until well mixed and the cereal and nuts are completely coated. Press the mixture into the prepared dish and refrigerate for about 1 hour until firm.

5. Cut the bars into 16 pieces and serve.

VARIATION TIP There are many types of nut butters available these days and any works in these charming treats. Try cashew butter, pecan butter, and even a more exotic macadamia butter for different flavors.

PER SERVING (2 pieces) Calories: 90; Total fat: 3g; Saturated fat: 0g; Carbohydrates: 17g; Fiber: 1g; Protein: 2g

BLACKBERRY-LEMON GRANITA

SERVES 4 **PREP** 10 minutes plus 4 hours to freeze

Granita is a semifrozen dessert that is a little like an adult slushy, but more spoon-friendly. If you do not own an ice-cream maker, you can still create an elegant dessert with a metal pan, fork, and lots of fresh fruit like the blackberries in this version. If your blackberries are very sweet and ripe, reduce the amount of honey in the dessert.

Make Ahead
Vegetarian

1 pound fresh blackberries

½ cup water

½ cup raw honey

¼ cup freshly squeezed lemon juice

1 teaspoon chopped fresh thyme

1. In a food processor, combine the blackberries, water, honey, lemon juice, and thyme. Pulse until puréed.

2. Pour the purée through a fine-mesh sieve into an 8-by-8-inch metal baking dish. Discard the seeds. Place the baking dish in the freezer for 2 hours. Remove the dish and stir the granita to break up any frozen sections, scraping along the sides. Return to the freezer for 1 hour. Stir and scrape again. Return the mixture to the freezer until completely frozen, about 4 hours total.

3. Cover the granita until you serve it. Use a fork to scrape off portions to serve.

SUBSTITUTION TIP Blackberries are a luscious fruit, sometimes the size of your thumb, bursting with sweetness and color. Other berries could be added to this recipe or used instead if your blackberries are not ripe enough. Try strawberries, raspberries, or blueberries in the same amount.

PER SERVING Calories: 182; Total fat: 1g; Saturated fat: 0g; Carbohydrates: 46g; Fiber: 6g; Protein: 2g

CLOVE-POACHED PEARS

SERVES 4 **PREP** 10 minutes **COOK** 15 minutes

Poached pears might seem like a lot of work, but the most time-consuming part is peeling the fruit. You are probably used to getting ripe fruit for your recipes, but in this case, you want the pears a little green so they don't fall apart when simmered. Don't worry that the pears might be a bit sour; they will be infused with honey.

Make Ahead
Vegetarian

4 cups water

2 cups unsweetened apple juice

¼ cup raw honey

1 teaspoon whole cloves

½ teaspoon whole cardamom seeds

1 teaspoon pure vanilla extract

4 pears, carefully peeled, halved lengthwise leaving the stem on one side, core removed

1. In a large saucepan over medium heat, combine the water, apple juice, honey, cloves, cardamom, and vanilla. Bring the mixture to a boil. Reduce the heat to low and simmer for 5 minutes.

2. Add the pear halves to the simmering liquid and cover the saucepan. Simmer the pears for about 10 minutes, turning several times until they are very tender.

3. With a slotted spoon, carefully remove the pears from the liquid and serve warm or cooled.

INGREDIENT TIP Pure vanilla extract has a rich flavor, but for the ultimate vanilla experience, use plump black Bourbon vanilla beans instead. Scrape the seeds from the pod directly into the simmering liquid, and add the empty pod as well.

PER SERVING Calories: 242; Total fat: 0g; Saturated fat: 0g; Carbohydrates: 63g; Fiber: 7g; Protein: 1g

TANGY LEMON MOUSSE

SERVES 4   **PREP** 10 minutes plus 2 hours to chill   **COOK** 4 minutes

Unless you are very experienced in the kitchen, you might not have used gelatin in any of your recipes. Gelatin is actually a very easy ingredient to use. Your results will be spectacular, as long as you follow a couple of simple rules: Never boil the gelatin mixture or it will not set, and use the gelatin mixture immediately after it is hydrated or it will congeal into a solid mass.

Make Ahead

¼ cup water

2 teaspoons powdered gelatin

2 cups canned lite coconut milk

½ cup freshly squeezed lemon juice

¼ cup raw honey

2 tablespoons freshly grated lemon zest

1. Put the water in a small saucepan. Sprinkle the gelatin over the water and set it aside for 10 minutes to soften.

2. In a medium bowl, whisk the coconut milk, lemon juice, honey, and lemon zest until well combined.

3. Place the saucepan with the gelatin over low heat. Gently heat the gelatin for about 4 minutes, or until just dissolved.

4. Whisk the gelatin mixture into the coconut milk mixture, and refrigerate for about 2 hours until set.

5. Scoop the lemon mousse into serving bowls.

VARIATION TIP Lemon is one of the most popular flavors in the world, but other citrus fruits can shine in this light and tangy dessert. Key limes can be used with no changes to the recipe, but if you wish to use oranges or grapefruit, cut the amount of honey in half.

PER SERVING Calories: 348; Total fat: 29g; Saturated fat: 25g; Carbohydrates: 25g; Fiber: 3g; Protein: 3g

LUSH PUMPKIN PUDDING

SERVES 6 **PREP** 10 minutes plus 2 hours to chill

Pecans add crunch and many health benefits to this creamy, rich, fall-themed dessert. Although most people call them nuts, pecans are actually the fruit of the pecan tree. Pecans are very high in phytonutrients, fiber, magnesium, copper, and phosphorus. Pecans can increase good (HDL) cholesterol and lower bad (LDL) cholesterol as well as support healthy cardiovascular and digestive systems.

Make Ahead

Vegan

2 cups canned full-fat coconut milk

1 cup pure pumpkin purée

¼ cup pure maple syrup

1 teaspoon ground cinnamon

½ teaspoon ground ginger

¼ teaspoon ground nutmeg

Pinch cloves

2 tablespoons chopped pecans, for garnish

1. In a large bowl, whisk the coconut milk, pumpkin, maple syrup, cinnamon, ginger, nutmeg, and cloves. Cover the bowl and refrigerator it for about 2 hours until chilled.

2. Serve topped with the pecans.

SUBSTITUTION TIP Sweet potato and butternut squash can be used here instead of pumpkin to create an equally delectable pudding. If nuts are an issue for you, omit the pecans as a garnish no matter which vegetable you choose.

PER SERVING Calories: 250; Total fat: 21g; Saturated fat: 17g; Carbohydrates: 17g; Fiber: 3g; Protein: 3g

SWEET GINGER PUDDING

SERVES 8 **PREP** 10 minutes **COOK** 50 minutes

Banana plays an important role in this traditional dessert. As well as providing sweetness and the moisture required to create the signature texture of cooked pudding, bananas are exceptionally high in potassium and are a wonderful source of fiber and vitamin B_6. This tropical fruit can help reduce digestive issues and support heart health.

Make Ahead

Vegetarian

½ cup coconut oil, at room temperature, plus more for greasing the baking dish

½ cup raw honey

1 banana

1 egg

2 teaspoons grated fresh ginger

1 teaspoon pure vanilla extract

2 cups almond flour

1 teaspoon baking soda

Pinch sea salt

1. Preheat the oven to 350°F.

2. Lightly grease an 8-by-8-inch baking dish with coconut oil and set it aside.

3. In a large bowl, beat the coconut oil, honey, banana, egg, ginger, and vanilla with a hand beater until well mixed, scraping down the sides of the bowl at least once.

4. Beat in the almond flour, baking soda, and sea salt. Spoon the batter into the prepared dish.

5. Bake for about 50 minutes, or until it is just set and lightly browned. Serve warm.

COOKING TIP Warm puddings were often steamed in large clean metal coffee cans. Although this pudding is not steamed, it can still be cooked in molds or coffee cans for a traditional look.

PREPARATION TIP You can also use a food processor to make this pudding, but pulse only a very few times to combine the ingredients.

PER SERVING Calories: 343; Total fat: 26g; Saturated fat: 13g; Carbohydrates: 26g; Fiber: 4g; Protein: 6g

BLUEBERRY-FIG OPEN-FACE PIE

SERVES 8 **PREP** 20 minutes plus 1 hour chilling **COOK** 30 minutes

Fruit pies are sometimes elaborate creations that look like they required hours of effort to create. Although lovely, an intricate-looking pie tastes identical to a simple open-face version featuring a couple cups of sweet fruit and about five minutes of rolling. You can change up the combination of fruit, but sweet figs combine beautifully with dark, delectable blueberries.

Make Ahead

Vegetarian

FOR THE CRUST

1¼ cups gluten-free flour

Pinch sea salt

⅓ cup chilled coconut oil, cut into ½-inch chunks

¼ cup ice water, or more as needed

TO MAKE THE CRUST

1. In a medium bowl, stir together the flour and sea salt.

2. Add the cold coconut oil. With a pastry blender or a fork, work the ingredients together until they form coarse crumbs.

3. Add the ice water, 1 tablespoon at a time, and stir with a fork until the dough just comes together. Transfer the dough to a sheet of plastic wrap and use your hands to firmly press the dough into a disk about ½ inch thick.

4. Wrap the dough tightly in plastic wrap and refrigerate for 1 hour until firm.

FOR THE FILLING

2 cups fresh blueberries

1 cup chopped fresh figs

¼ cup raw honey

1 tablespoon
arrowroot powder

¼ teaspoon ground nutmeg

1 egg, beaten

TO MAKE THE FILLING

1. Preheat the oven to 350°F.

2. Line a baking sheet with parchment paper and set it aside.

3. In a large bowl, toss together the blueberries, figs, honey, arrowroot powder, and nutmeg. Set it aside.

4. Place a sheet of wax paper on a work surface, and place the unwrapped dough in the center. Cover the dough with another sheet of wax paper, and gently roll it into a circle about 12 inches in diameter. Transfer the crust to the parchment-lined sheet.

5. Pour the berry mixture into the center of the crust. Spread out the berries, leaving about 1½ inches of empty crust around the edges.

6. Brush the empty crust with the beaten egg. Fold the edges of the crust over a bit of the filling, pressing lightly so the overlapping pieces of pastry stick together. Don't worry if it breaks; just patch it back together.

7. Bake the pie for about 30 minutes, or until the crust is golden and crisp and the filling is bubbling.

COOKING TIP Arrange this piecrust in a fluted mold or in a traditional pie plate if free form does not suit your needs. A gluten-free crust can be crumbly, so take care when sliding it into the pan.

PER SERVING Calories: 237; Total fat: 9g; Saturated fat: 8g; Carbohydrates: 38g; Fiber: 2g; Protein: 2g

BERRY-RHUBARB COBBLER

SERVES 8 **PREP** 15 minutes **COOK** 35 minutes

Rhubarb is an incredible vegetable to grow in your garden (if you have the space) because it thrives without any special treatment. This recipe treats rhubarb like a fruit, combining it with berries and a sweet coconut-almond topping. Rhubarb is a stellar source of vitamin K, lutein, and calcium. Make sure you use only the stems; cut off the leaves and discard them because they are toxic.

Make Ahead

Vegetarian

FOR THE COBBLER

Coconut oil, for greasing the baking dish

2 cups fresh blueberries

1 cup fresh raspberries

1 cup sliced (½-inch) rhubarb pieces

¼ cup unsweetened apple juice

¼ cup raw honey

1 tablespoon arrowroot powder

FOR THE TOPPING

1 cup almond flour

½ cup shredded unsweetened coconut

1 tablespoon arrowroot powder

½ cup coconut oil

¼ cup raw honey

TO MAKE THE COBBLER

1. Preheat the oven to 350°F.

2. Lightly grease a 9-by-9-inch baking dish with coconut oil and set it aside.

3. In a large bowl, toss together the blueberries, raspberries, rhubarb, apple juice, honey, and arrowroot powder until combined. Transfer the fruit mixture to the prepared dish and spread it out evenly.

TO MAKE THE TOPPING

1. In a small bowl, stir together the almond flour, coconut, and arrowroot powder until well mixed.

2. Add the coconut oil and honey. With a fork, mix until coarse crumbs form. Spread the topping on top of the fruit in the baking dish.

3. Bake the crumble for about 35 minutes, or until bubbly and golden.

VARIATION TIP As with many other fruit desserts, you can change up the fruit filling for this cobbler easily, using the same amounts for the new ingredients. Peaches, plums, cherries, apples, pears—even sweet potato and pumpkin—make marvelous options depending on the season and availability of the produce.

PER SERVING Calories: 304; Total fat: 22g; Saturated fat: 14g; Carbohydrates: 30g; Fiber: 4g; Protein: 3g

TENDER COCONUT CAKE

SERVES 8 **PREP** 15 minutes **COOK** 45 minutes

Whenever possible, use fresh coconut in your recipes because it tastes infinitely better than desiccated products. Cracking a coconut is not as hard as you think; just use the blunt side of a chef's knife to strike the coconut all the way around the perimeter. Do this over a bowl to collect the water when the coconut breaks open. Simply pry the meat away from the shell and grate it for your recipes.

Make Ahead

Vegetarian

½ cup coconut oil, melted, plus more for greasing the baking dish

2 cups egg whites (about 12), at room temperature

Pinch sea salt

1 cup unsweetened almond milk

6 tablespoons raw honey

2 teaspoons pure vanilla extract

1 cup coconut flour

½ cup shredded unsweetened coconut

2 teaspoons baking powder

1. Preheat the oven to 350°F.

2. Lightly grease a 9-by-13-inch baking dish with coconut oil and set it aside.

3. In a large bowl, beat the egg whites and sea salt with an electric mixer until soft peaks form. Set them aside.

4. In another large bowl, whisk the almond milk, honey, remaining ½ cup of coconut oil, and the vanilla.

5. Whisk in the coconut flour, coconut, and baking powder until well combined.

6. Fold the beaten egg whites into the batter, keeping as much volume as possible, until just blended. Spoon the batter into the prepared dish and smooth the top.

7. Bake the cake for about 45 minutes, or until cooked through and lightly browned.

8. Cool the cake completely on a wire rack.

9. Serve with fresh fruit, if desired.

SUBSTITUTION TIP For an entirely coconut-flavored cake, swap the almond milk for the same quantity of unsweetened coconut milk. There is a taste difference you will notice between the two nondairy milk products.

PER SERVING Calories: 237; Total fat: 17g; Saturated fat: 15g; Carbohydrates: 16g; Fiber: 1g; Protein: 7g

MAPLE CARROT CAKE

SERVES 12 **PREP** 15 minutes **COOK** 45 minutes

Carrot cake is a lovely choice for a birthday or special event, especially when warmly spiced with cinnamon and nutmeg. Finely ground coconut flour creates a tender crumb, so you need to cool the cake sufficiently as the finished product can be a little crumbly and delicate when still warm. If you want an even more striking contrast, grate the carrot more coarsely and add a little shredded coconut as well.

Make Ahead

Vegetarian

½ cup coconut oil, at room temperature, plus more for greasing the baking dish

¼ cup pure maple syrup

2 teaspoons pure vanilla extract

6 eggs

½ cup coconut flour

1 teaspoon baking soda

1 teaspoon baking powder

1 teaspoon ground cinnamon

½ teaspoon ground nutmeg

⅛ teaspoon sea salt

3 cups finely grated carrots

½ cup chopped pecans

1. Preheat the oven to 350°F.

2. Lightly grease a 9-by-13-inch baking dish with coconut oil and set it aside.

3. In a large bowl, whisk the ½ cup of coconut oil, maple syrup, and vanilla until blended.

4. One at a time, whisk in the eggs, beating well after each addition.

5. In a medium bowl, stir together the coconut flour, baking soda, baking powder, cinnamon, nutmeg, and sea salt. Add the dry ingredients to the wet ingredients, and stir until just combined.

6. Stir in the carrots and pecans until mixed. Spoon the batter into the prepared dish.

7. Bake for about 45 minutes, or until a toothpick inserted in the center comes out clean.

8. Cool the cake on a wire rack and serve.

SUBSTITUTION TIP Pecans combine beautifully with the moist, sweet carrot and warm spices of this cake. However, leave this rich tree nut out if there is any concern about nut allergies.

PER SERVING Calories: 254; Total fat: 21g; Saturated fat: 15g; Carbohydrates: 13g; Fiber: 2g; Protein: 5g

RICH CAROB SHEET CAKE

SERVES 12 **PREP** 10 minutes **COOK** 40 minutes

This tender cake uses a substantial amount of coconut oil, which might make you think the portions are too high in fat. Although coconut oil is high in saturated fat, it is mostly medium-chain triglycerides, unlike animal fats, which are long-chain fats. This means it is synthesized directly in the liver and converted to energy rather than deposited as fat like other types of saturated fat.

Make Ahead

Vegetarian

1 cup melted coconut oil, plus more for greasing the baking dish

10 eggs

1 cup pure maple syrup

2 teaspoons pure vanilla extract

¾ cup coconut flour

½ cup carob powder

1 teaspoon baking soda

⅛ teaspoon sea salt

1. Preheat the oven to 350°F.

2. Lightly grease a 9-by-13-inch baking dish with coconut oil and set it aside.

3. In a large bowl, beat or whisk the eggs until frothy.

4. Add the remaining 1 cup of coconut oil, the maple syrup, and vanilla. Beat or whisk until well blended.

5. In a small bowl, stir together the coconut flour, carob powder, baking soda, and sea salt. Add the dry ingredients to the wet ingredients and blend until smooth. Pour the batter into the prepared dish.

6. Bake for about 40 minutes, or until a knife inserted in the center comes out clean.

7. Remove the cake from the oven and let it cool on a wire rack.

8. Serve with fruit or topped with whipped coconut cream, if desired.

VARIATION TIP Chocolate glaze is the perfect finish for this cake and is easy to make. In a small saucepan over low heat, whisk ½ cup of carob powder and ½ cup of unsweetened almond milk until smooth. Whisk in 2 tablespoons of raw honey and 1 teaspoon of pure vanilla extract. Pour the glaze over the cake and refrigerate for 30 minutes.

PER SERVING Calories: 312; Total fat: 25g; Saturated fat: 19g; Carbohydrates: 21g; Fiber: 2g; Protein: 6g

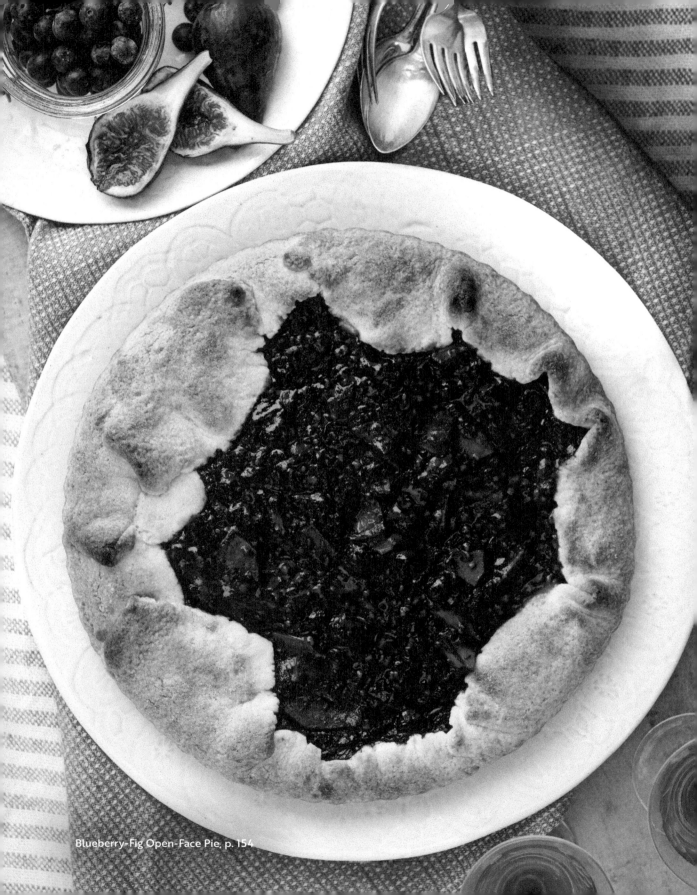

Blueberry-Fig Open-Face Pie, p. 154

APPENDIX A
THE RHEUMATOID ARTHRITIS DIET MEAL PLANS

As mentioned in chapter 1 (page 17), weight loss is not as simple as "calories in, calories out." The quality of our food matters, and reducing inflammation in the body is important for a weight management goal. However, this is not to say calories do not matter at all. It can be helpful to track your calorie intake when you have a specific weight goal in mind.

To do this, calculate your basal metabolic rate (BMR), which is the amount of calories your body needs to function at rest. Your BMR takes into consideration your age and weight. Adjust this based on your daily activity level. You can find BMR calculators online, such as the Mayo Clinic's Calorie Calculator (www.mayoclinic.org/diseases-conditions/obesity/in-depth/bmi-calculator/itt-20084938), or you can use a food-tracking app, such as MyFitnessPal (www.myfitnesspal.com), that will calculate this for you.

A healthy weight loss is ½ to 2 pounds per week. This is a gradual, safe weight loss. To lose 1 pound per week, you need to reduce your calorie intake by 3,500 calories for the week. This would be a calorie deficit of 500 calories per day, which you could do through both nutrition and exercise (reduce 250 calories in the diet and burn 250 calories through exercise).

Let's assume you want to create this calorie deficit through nutrition alone. After you calculate your BMR, subtract 500 calories from this number to get your daily calorie target for a one-pound-per-week loss. For example:

- Your BMR is 1,900 calories per day.

- You want to lose 1 pound per week.

- Subtract 500 calories (for a total of 3,500 for the week).

- Your daily calorie goal is 1,400 calories.

If weight gain is your goal and you want to do this at a rate of ½ pound per week, add 250 calories (for a weekly total of 1,750 additional calories) to your BMR calculation for your daily calorie goal. Keep in mind that you want to achieve weight gain with good-quality food.

The following meal plans are based on a 1,600-calorie-per-day diet that takes snacks into account. You may need to increase or decrease the calories based on your goal and current BMR. The plans contain nutritious anti-inflammatory foods that support your body to help you achieve your goal. I also recommend food tracking with an app to help monitor your calories for the day.

WEEK ONE MEAL PLAN

Monday

Breakfast: Apple-Honey Smoothie (page 40)

Lunch: Green Mango Slaw with Cashews (page 92)

Dinner: Baked Halibut with Avocado Salsa (page 125) and Buckwheat Tabbouleh (double recipe, page 69)

Tuesday

Breakfast: Fruit-and-Seed Breakfast Bars (page 41)

Lunch: Chilled Coconut-Avocado Soup (double recipe, page 85)

Dinner: Grainy Mustard–Crusted Lamb (page 140) and Buckwheat Tabbouleh (leftovers)

Wednesday

Breakfast: Creamy Pistachio Smoothie (page 37)

Lunch: Chilled Coconut-Avocado Soup (leftovers)

Dinner: Herb-Roasted Chicken (page 132) and Coconut-Almond Bake (page 73)

Thursday

Breakfast: Egg Casserole with Sweet Potato and Kale (page 45)

Lunch: Artichoke-Almond Salad (page 98)

Dinner: Buckwheat Burgers (double recipe, page 113) and Shredded Root Vegetable Salad (double recipe, page 97)

Friday

Breakfast: Mini Broccoli Frittatas (page 44)

Lunch: Buckwheat Burgers (leftovers), Shredded Root Vegetable Salad (leftovers)

Dinner: Beef Sirloin Kebabs in Garlic Marinade (page 143) and Seasoned Carrot Batons (page 64)

Saturday

Breakfast: Golden Coconut Pancakes (page 43)

Lunch: Classic French Onion Soup (double, recipe page 81)

Dinner: Coconut-Braised Chicken (page 133) and Wild Rice–Stuffed Sweet Potatoes (page 112)

Sunday

Breakfast: "Chocolate"-Avocado Smoothie (page 35)

Lunch: Classic French Onion Soup (leftovers)

Dinner: Coconut Milk–Baked Sole (page 122), Sautéed Kale with Garlic (page 68), and Vegetable Quinoa (page 72)

Suggested Snacks

Rich Carob Sheet Cake (page 159)

Cucumber slices with Avocado-Herb Spread (page 55)

Hardboiled eggs or nitrite- and nitrate-free sliced turkey with carrot sticks

Watermelon or cantaloupe

Crudités

Good-quality grass-fed beef or turkey bar (such as Epic Bar) paired with a vegetable, for example, celery sticks

WEEK TWO MEAL PLAN

Monday

Breakfast: Minty Green Smoothie (page 36)

Lunch: Mushroom Egg Foo Young (page 104)

Dinner: Chicken Buckwheat Florentine (double recipe, page 134)

Tuesday

Breakfast: Fruit-and-Seed Breakfast Bars (page 41)

Lunch: Chicken Buckwheat Florentine (leftovers)

Dinner: Pork Loin with Roasted Fennel and Celeriac (page 139) and Wild Rice–Cauliflower Pilaf (page 70)

Wednesday

Breakfast: Sweet Potato Pie Smoothie (page 39)

Lunch: Beef and Vegetable Soup (double recipe, page 89)

Dinner: Spice-Rubbed Salmon with Tangerine Relish (page 124) and Broccoli Salad with Rainier Cherry Dressing (page 100)

Thursday

Breakfast: Mini Broccoli Frittatas (page 44)

Lunch: Beef and Vegetable Soup (leftovers)

Dinner: Pumpkin Curry (double recipe, page 111) and Buckwheat Tabbouleh (page 69)

Friday

Breakfast: Tropical Red Smoothie (page 38)

Lunch: Pumpkin Curry (leftovers)

Dinner: Turkey-Thyme Meatballs (page 135) and Vegetable Quinoa (page 72)

Saturday

Breakfast: Golden Coconut Pancakes (page 43) with honey and fresh berries

Lunch: Thai Cabbage Bowl (page 109)

Dinner: Coconut Crab Cakes (double recipe, page 117) and Artichoke-Almond Salad (page 98)

Sunday

Breakfast: Egg Casserole with Sweet Potato and Kale (page 45)

Lunch: Coconut Crab Cakes (leftovers)

Dinner: Pork Chops with Cooked Apple Salsa (page 138) and Caramelized Celeriac (page 66)

Suggested Snacks

Fruit-and-Seed Breakfast Bars (page 41)

Sweet Carrot Spread (page 57) wrapped in a romaine lettuce leaf

Fresh berries

Celery or apple with almond butter

1 serving of nuts (¼ cup) such as cashews

Good-quality turkey or beef jerky, such as from The New Primal paired with a vegetable, for example, sugar snap peas

Green or black olives with a few slices of nitrite/nitrate-free salami and a pickle (yellow dye- and preservative-free)

CONVERSION TABLES

Volume Equivalents (Liquid)

US STANDARD	US STANDARD (OUNCES)	METRIC (APPROXIMATE)
2 tablespoons	1 fl. oz.	30 mL
¼ cup	2 fl. oz.	60 mL
½ cup	4 fl. oz.	120 mL
1 cup	8 fl. oz.	240 mL
1½ cups	12 fl. oz.	355 mL
2 cups or 1 pint	16 fl. oz.	475 mL
4 cups or 1 quart	32 fl. oz.	1 L
1 gallon	128 fl. oz.	4 L

Oven Temperatures

FAHRENHEIT	CELSIUS (APPROXIMATE)
250°F	120°C
300°F	150°C
325°F	165°C
350°F	180°C
375°F	190°C
400°F	200°C
425°F	220°C
450°F	230°C

Volume Equivalents (Dry)

US STANDARD	METRIC (APPROXIMATE)
⅛ teaspoon	0.5 mL
¼ teaspoon	1 mL
½ teaspoon	2 mL
¾ teaspoon	4 mL
1 teaspoon	5 mL
1 tablespoon	15 mL
¼ cup	59 mL
⅓ cup	79 mL
½ cup	118 mL
⅔ cup	156 mL
¾ cup	177 mL
1 cup	235 mL
2 cups or 1 pint	475 mL
3 cups	700 mL
4 cups or 1 quart	1 L

Weight Equivalents

US STANDARD	METRIC (APPROXIMATE)
½ ounce	15 g
1 ounce	30 g
2 ounces	60 g
4 ounces	115 g
8 ounces	225 g
12 ounces	340 g
16 ounces or 1 pound	455 g

THE DIRTY DOZEN & THE CLEAN FIFTEEN

A nonprofit environmental watchdog organization called Environmental Working Group (EWG) looks at data supplied by the U.S. Department of Agriculture (USDA) and the Food and Drug Administration (FDA) about pesticide residues. Each year it compiles a list of the best and worst pesticide loads found in commercial crops. You can use these lists to decide which fruits and vegetables to buy organic to minimize your exposure to pesticides, and which produce is considered safe enough to buy conventionally. This does not mean they are pesticide-free, though, so wash these fruits and vegetables thoroughly.

These lists change every year, so make sure you look up the most recent one before you fill your shopping cart. You'll find the most recent lists, as well as a guide to pesticides in produce, at EWG.org/FoodNews.

DIRTY DOZEN

Apples	Strawberries
Celery	Sweet bell peppers
Cherries	Tomatoes
Cherry tomatoes	*In addition to the Dirty*
Cucumbers	*Dozen, the EWG added*
Grapes	*two types of produce*
Nectarines	*contaminated with highly*
Peaches	*toxic organophosphate*
Spinach	*insecticides:*
	Kale/Collard greens
	Hot peppers

CLEAN FIFTEEN

Asparagus	Kiwis
Avocados	Mangos
Cabbage	Onions
Cantaloupe	Papayas
Cauliflower	Pineapples
Eggplant	Sweet corn
Grapefruit	Sweet peas (frozen)
Honeydew Melon	

RESOURCES

Explore the resources here for more information on managing and living with your arthritis.

Websites

Arthritis Foundation:
www.arthritis.org

The Autoimmune Protocol:
https://aiplifestyle.com

Book on Natural RA Treatments

Kamhi, Ellen, and Eugene Zampieron. *Alternative Medicine Definitive Guide to Arthritis: Reverse Underlying Causes of Arthritis with Clinically Proven Alternative Therapies.* 2nd ed. Berkeley, CA: Celestial Arts, 2006

Support Groups for Young and Middle-Aged Adults with RA

Arthritis Introspective:
www.arthritisintrospective.org

Local resources for RA support from the Arthritis Foundation:
http://resourcefinder.arthritis.org/?_ga=
1.238532032.1778446959.1
446493347

App for Managing RA

The Arthritis Foundation's Arthritis Tracker, Track + React, helps on a daily basis and includes recording sleep, food, exercise, pain levels, and medications:
www.arthritis.org/living-with-arthritis
/tools-resources/track-and-react/

Blog

From This Point Forward:
www.fromthispointforward.com

Magazine

Arthritis Today

REFERENCES

Ajibola, A., J. P. Chamunorwa, and K. H. Erlwanger. "Nutraceutical Values of Natural Honey and Its Contribution to Human Health and Wealth." *Nutrition and Metabolism* 9, no. 61 (June 2012). doi:10.1186/1743-7075-9-61.

American Heart Association. "Sugar 101." Accessed November 20, 2016. www.heart.org/HEARTORG/HealthyLiving/HealthyEating/HealthyDietGoals/Sugar-101_UCM_306024_Article.jsp#.WDTnd3jhoy8.

American Heart Association. "Suggested Servings from Each Food Group." Accessed December 11, 2016. www.heart.org/HEARTORG/HealthyLiving/HealthyEating/Nutrition/Suggested-Servings-from-Each-Food-Group_UCM_318186_Article.jsp#.WFIHk3jhoy8.

Appleton, Nancy. *Lick the Sugar Habit.* Garden City Park, NY: Avery, 1996.

Arthritis Foundation. "Corticosteroid Use in Rheumatoid Arthritis." Accessed November 6, 2016. www.arthritis.org/living-with-arthritis/treatments/medication/drug-types/corticosteroids/ra-corticosteroid.php.

Arthritis Foundation. "DMARDs Overview." Accessed November 6, 2016. www.arthritis.org/living-with-arthritis/treatments/medication/drug-types/disease-modifying-drugs/drug-guide-dmards.php.

Arthritis Foundation. "NSAIDs." Accessed November 6, 2016. www.arthritis.org/living-with-arthritis/treatments/medication/drug-guide/drug-class/nsaids.php.

Arthritis Foundation. "Rheumatoid Arthritis Causes." Accessed November 6, 2016. www.arthritis.org/about-arthritis/types/rheumatoid-arthritis/causes.php.

Arthritis Foundation. "Rheumatoid Arthritis Treatment." Accessed November 6, 2016. www.arthritis.org/about-arthritis/types/rheumatoid-arthritis/treatment.php.

Beauchamp, G. K., R. S. Keast, D. Morel, et al. "Phytochemistry: Ibuprofen-Like Activity in Extra-Virgin Olive Oil." *Nature* 437 (September 2005): 45–6. doi:10.1038/437045a.

Benelam, B., and L. Wyness. "Hydration and Health: A Review." *Nutrition Bulletin* 35, no. 1 (March 2010): 3–25. doi:10.1111/j.1467-3010.2009.01795.x.

Calder, P. C. "Immunoregulatory and Anti-Inflammatory Effects of N-3 Polyunsaturated Fatty Acids." *Brazilian Journal of Medical and Biological Research* 31, no. 4 (April 1998): 467–490. doi.org/10.1590/S0100-879X1998000400002.

Cantor, M. T., and B. D. Mahon. "Mounting Evidence for Vitamin D as an Environmental Factor Affecting Autoimmune Disease Prevalence." *Experimental Biology and Medicine* 229, no. 11 (December 2004): 1136–1142. PMID: 15564440.

Carman, J. A., H. R. Vlieger, L. J. Ver Steeg, et al. "A Long-Term Toxicology Study on Pigs Fed a Combined Genetically Modified (GM) Soy and GM Maize Diet, Associated with Weight Gain and Severe Stomach Inflammation." *Journal of Organic Systems* 8, no. 1 (June 2013): 38–54.

Centers for Disease Control. "Rheumatoid Arthritis." Accessed November 6, 2016. www.cdc.gov/arthritis/basics/rheumatoid .htm.

Cortes-Rojas, D. F., C. R. Fernandes de Souza, and W. P. Oliveira. "Clove (Syzygium Aromaticum): A Precious Spice." *Asian Pacific Journal of Tropical Biomedicine* 4, no. 2 (February 2014): 90–96. doi:10.1016/S2221-1691(14)60215-X.

Covington, M. B. "Omega-3 Fatty Acids." *American Family Physician* 70, no. 1 (July 2004): 133–140. PMID: 15259529.

Cusick, M. F., J. E. Libbey, and R. S. Fujinami. "Molecular Mimicry as a Mechanism of Autoimmune Disease." *Clinical Reviews in Allergy and Immunology* 42, no. 1 (February 2012): 102–111. doi:10.1007 /s12016-011-8294-7.

Daley, C. A., A. Abbott, P. S. Doyle, G. A. Nader, and S. Larson. "A Review of Fatty Acid Profiles and Antioxidant Content in Grass-Fed and Grain-Fed Beef." *Nutrition Journal* 9, no. 10 (March 2010). doi:10.1186/1475-2891-9-10.

DeChristopher, L. R., J. Uribarri, and K. L. Tucker. "Intake of High-Fructose Corn Syrup Sweetened Soft Drinks, Fruit Drinks, and Apple Juice Is Associated with Prevalent Arthritis in U.S. Adults, Aged 20–30 Years. *Nutrition and Diabetes* 6, no. e199 (March 2016). doi:10.1038/nutd.2016.7.

Domingo, J. L. "Omega-3 Fatty Acids and the Benefits of Fish Consumption: Is All That Glitters Gold?" *Environment International* 33, no. 7 (October 2007): 993–998. doi:10.1152/ajpheart.01104.2006.

Dupasquier, C. M., E. Dibrov, A.L. Kneesh, et al. "Dietary Flaxseed Inhibits Atherosclerosis in the LDL Receptor-Deficient Mouse in Part Through Antiproliferative and Anti-Inflammatory Actions." *American Journal of Physiology— Heart and Circulatory Physiology* 293, no. 4 (October 2007): H2394–402. doi:10.1152/ajpheart.01104.2006.

Enbrel. "Benefits vs. Risks: What to Know about the Side Effects of Enbrel." Accessed December 12, 2016. www.enbrel.com /support/side-effects-safety-information/.

Environmental Protection Agency. "EPA-FDA Advisory on Mercury in Fish and Shellfish." Accessed November 20, 2016. www.epa.gov/fish-tech/epa-fda -advisory-mercury-fish-and-shellfish.

Esmaillzadeh, A., M. Kimiagar, Y. Mehrabi, et al. "Fruit and Vegetable Intakes, C-Reactive Protein, and the Metabolic Syndrome." *American Journal of Clinical Nutrition* 84, no. 6 (December 2006): 1489–1497. PMID: 17158434.

Fallon, Sally, and Mary G. Enig. *Nourishing Traditions: The Cookbook that Challenges Politically Correct Nutrition and the Diet Dictocrats.* Brandywine, MD: New Trends Publishing, 2001.

Festa, A., R. D'Agostino Jr., K. Williams, et al. "The Relation of Body Fat Mass and Distribution to Markers of Chronic Inflammation." *International Journal of Obesity and Related Metabolic Disorders* 25, no. 10 (October 2001): 1407–15. doi:10.1038/sj.ijo.0801792.

Food Insight. "New Dietary Guidelines: What Changed and What Stayed the Same." Accessed November 20, 2016. www.foodinsight.org/new-dietary-guidelines-americans-2015-changes#Cholestorol.

Fretts, A. M., B. V. Howard, B. McKnight, et al. "Associations of Processed Meat and Unprocessed Red Meat Intake with Incident Diabetes: The Strong Heart Family Study." *American Journal of Clinical Nutrition* 95, no. 3 (March 2012): 752–758. doi:10.3945/ajcn.111.029942.

Frost, Mary. *Back to the Basics of Human Health: Avoiding the Fads, Trends, and Bold-Faced Lies.* San Diego, CA: Expansive Health Awareness, Inc. 2010.

Gabriel, S. E. "The Epidemiology of Rheumatoid Arthritis." *Rheumatic Disease Clinics of North America* 27, no. 2 (May 2001): 269–8. PMID: 11396092.

Grzanna, R., L. Lindmark, and C. G. Frondoza. "Ginger—An Herbal Medicinal Product with Broad Anti-Inflammatory Actions." *Journal of Medicinal Food* 8, no. 2 (July 2005): 125–132. doi:10.1089/jmf.2005.8.125.

Healthline. "Find the Best Medications for Rheumatoid Arthritis." Accessed November 6, 2016. www.healthline.com/health/consumer-reports-rheumatoid-arthritis.

Holyoke, M. F., and T. C. Chen. "Vitamin D Deficiency: A Worldwide Problem with Health Consequences." *American Journal of Clinical Nutrition* 87, no. 4 (April 2008): 1080S–1086S. PMID: 18400738.

Huang, W. Y., Y. Z. Cai, and Y. Zhang. "Natural Phenolic Compounds from Medicinal Herbs and Dietary Plants: Potential Use for Cancer Prevention." *Nutrition and Cancer* 62, no. 1 (2010): 1–20. doi:10.1080/01635580903191585.

Humira. "Frequently Asked Questions about Humira." Accessed December 12, 2016. www.humira.com/global/frequently-asked-questions.

Hvatum, M., L. Kanerud, R. Hällgren, and P. Brandtzaeg. "The Gut-Joint Axis: Cross-Reactive Food Antibodies in Rheumatoid Arthritis" *Gut* 55, no. 9 (September 2006): 1240–1247. doi:10.1136/gut.2005.076901.

Johnson, R.J., M. S. Segal, Y. Sautin, et al. "Potential Role of Sugar (Fructose) in the Epidemic of Hypertension, Obesity, and the Metabolic Syndrome, Diabetes, Kidney Disease, and Cardiovascular Disease." *American Journal of Clinical Nutrition* 86, no. 4 (October 2007): 899–906. http://ajcn.nutrition.org/content/86/4/899.full.

Joseph, S. V., I. Edirisinghe, and B. M. Burton-Freeman. "Berries: Anti-Inflammatory Effects in Humans." *Journal of Agriculture and Food Chemistry* 62, no. 18 (May 2014): 3886–903. doi:10.1021/jf4044056.

Kamhi, E., and E. R. Zampieron. *Alternative Medicine Definitive Guide to Arthritis: Reverse Underlying Causes of Arthritis with Clinically Proven Alternative Therapies.* 2nd ed. Berkeley, CA: Celestial Arts, 2006.

Katan, M. B. "Nitrate in Foods: Harmful or Healthy?" *American Journal of Clinical Nutrition* 90, no. 1 (July 2009): doi:10.3945/ajcn.2009.28014.

King'ori, A. M. "Influence of Poultry Diet on the Fatty Acid, Mineral, and Vitamin Composition of the Egg: A Review." *Journal of Animal Science Advances* 2, no. 7 (2012): 583–588. www.scopemed.org/?jft=72&ft=72-1340889312.

Liu, H., J. C. Schmitz, J. Wei, et al. "Clove Extract Inhibits Tumor Growth and Promotes Cell Cycle Arrest and Apoptosis." *Oncology Research* 21, no. 5 (2014): 247–259. doi:10.3727/096504014X13946388748910.

Lopez-Garcia, E., M. B. Schulze, J. B. Meigs, et al. "Consumption of Trans Fatty Acids Is Related to Plasma Biomarkers of Inflammation and Endothelial Dysfunction." *The Journal of Nutrition* 135, no. 3 (March 2005): 562–566. PMID: 15735094.

Manzel, A., D. N. Muller, D.A. Hafler, et al. "Role of 'Western Diet' in Inflammatory Autoimmune Diseases." *Current Allergy Asthma Reports* 14, no. 1 (January 2014): 404. doi:10.1007/s11882-013-0404-6.

Margaretten, M., L. Julian, P. Katz, and E. Yellin. "Depression in Patients with Rheumatoid Arthritis: Description, Causes, and Mechanisms." *International Journal of Clinical Rheumatology* 6, no. 6 (December 2011): 617–623. doi:10.2217/IJR.11.6

Matcham, F., L. Rayner, S. Steer, and M. Hotopf. "The Prevalence of Depression in Rheumatoid Arthritis: A Systematic Review and Meta-Analysis." *Rheumatology* 52, no. 12 (December 2013): 2136–48. doi:10.1093/rheumatology/ket169.

McAfee, A. J., E. M. McSorley, G. J. Cuskelly, et al. "Red Meat from Animals Offered a Grass Diet Increases Plasma and Platelet N-3 PUFA in Healthy Consumers." *British Journal of Nutrition* 105, no. 1 (January 2011): 80–9. doi:10.1017/S0007114510003090.

Mercola. "Nine Things Everyone Should Know about Farmed Fish." Accessed November 20, 2016. http://articles.mercola.com/sites/articles/archive/2013/12/21/9-farmed-fish-facts.aspx.

Miles, E. A., P. Zoubouli, and P. C. Calder. "Differential Anti-Inflammatory Effects of Phenolic Compounds from Extra-Virgin Olive Oil Identified in Human Whole Blood Cultures." *Nutrition* 21, no. 3 (March 2005): 389–394. doi:10.1016/j.nut.2004.06.031.

Momtazi-Borojeni, A. A., S. A. Esmaeili, E. Abdollahi, and A. Sahebkar. "A Review on the Pharmacology and Toxicology of Steviol Glycosides Extracted from Stevia Rebaudiana." *Current Pharmaceutical Design* 22 (October 2016): doi:10.2174/13816 12822666161021142835.

Nettleton, J. A. "Fatty Acids in Cultivated and Wild Fish. Microbehavior and Macroresults." *Proceedings of the Tenth Biennial Conference of the International Institute of Fisheries Economics and Trade.* July 10–14, 2000. Compiled by Richard S. Johnston and Ann L. Shriver. Corvallis, OR: International Institute of Fisheries Economics and Trade, 2001.

Obesity Society. "U.S. Adult Consumption of Added Sugars Increased by More Than 30 percent over Three Decades." Accessed November 20, 2016. www.obesity.org /news/press-releases/us-adult.

Pallavi, K., and R. Rajagopalan. "Cinnamon: Mystic Powers of a Minute Ingredient." *Pharmacognosy Research* 7, Supplement 1 (June 2015): S1–S6. doi:10.4103/0974-8490.157990.

Pandey, K. B., and S. I. Rizvi. "Plant Polyphenols as Dietary Antioxidants in Human Health and Disease." *Oxidative Medicine and Cellular Longevity* 2, no. 5 (November–December 2009): 270–278. doi:10.4161/oxim.2.5.9498.

Qi, S., R. Xin, W. Guo, and Y. Liu. "Meta-Analysis of Oral Contraceptives and Rheumatoid Arthritis Risk in Women." *Journal of Therapeutics and Clinical Risk Management* 10 (November 2014): 915–923. doi:10.2147/TCRM.S70867.

Ramsewak, R. S., D. L. DeWitt, and M. G. Nair. "Cytotoxicity, Antioxidant, and Anti-Inflammatory Activities of Curcumins 1-111 from *Curcuma Longa*." *Phytomedicine* 7, no. 4 (July 2000): 303–308. doi:10.1016/S0944-7113(00)80048-3.

Rivlin, R. S. "Recent Advances on the Nutritional Effects Associated with the Use of Garlic as a Supplement." *Journal of Nutrition* 131 (2001): 951S–954S. http://jn.nutrition.org/content/131 /3/951S.full.pdf.

Roubenoff, R. "Sarcopenic Obesity: Does Muscle Loss Cause Fat Gain? Lessons from Rheumatoid Arthritis and Osteoarthritis." *Annals of the New York Academy of Sciences* 904, no. 1 (May 2000): 553–7. PMID: 10865804.

Sapone, A., J. C. Bai, C. Ciacci, et al. "Spectrum of Gluten-Related Disorders: Consensus on New Nomenclature and Classification." *BMC Medicine* 10, no. 13 (February 2012). doi:10.1186/1741-7015-10-13.

Schrezenmeir, J., and M. de Vrese. "Probiotics, Prebiotics, and Synbiotics—Approaching a Definition." *American Journal of Clinical Nutrition* 73, no. 2 (February 2001): 361s–364s. http://ajcn.nutrition.org/content/73/2/361s.full.pdf+html.

Snack Works. "Nabisco 100-Calorie Packs Oreo Thin Crisps 0.81 Oz." Accessed November 6, 2016. www.snackworks.com/products/product-detail.aspx?product=4400000617.

Taneja, V. "Arthritis Susceptibility and the Gut Microbiome." *FEBS Letters* 588, no. 22 (November 2014): 4244–9. doi:10.1016/j.febslet.2014.05.034.

Thacher, T. D., and B. L. Clarke. "Vitamin D Insufficiency." *Mayo Clinic Proceedings* 86, no. 1 (January 2011): 50–60. doi:10.4065/mcp.2010.0567.

Tipoe, G. L., T. M. Leung, M. W. Hung, and M. L. Fung. "Green Tea Polyphenols as an Anti-Oxidant and Anti-Inflammatory Agent for Cardiovascular Protection." *Cardiovascular and Hematological Disorders Drug Targets* 7, no. 2 (June 2007): 135–44. PMID: 17584048.

Tobón, G. J., P. Youinou, and A. Saraux. "The Environment, Geo-Epidemiology, and Autoimmune Disease: Rheumatoid Arthritis." *Journal of Autoimmunity* 35, no. 1 (August 2010): 10–14. doi:10.1016/j.jaut.2009.12.009.

Vagnini, F. J., and Barry Fox. *The Side Effects Bible: The Dietary Solution to Unwanted Side Effects of Common Medications.* New York: Broadway, 2005.

Virgin, J.J. "Good Morning America Crushes Womens' Motivation to Exercise." Accessed November 20, 2016. http://jjvirgin.com/good-morning-america-crushes-womens-motivation-to-exercise/

Vojdani, A., and I. Tarash. "Cross-Reaction between Gliadin and Different Food and Tissue Antigens." *Food and Nutrition Sciences* 4, no. 1 (January 2013): 20–32. doi:10.4236/fns.2013.41005.

Vysakh, A., M. Ratheesh, T. P. Rajmohanan, et al. "Polyphenolics Isolated from Virgin Coconut Oil Inhibits Adjuvant Induced Arthritis in Rats through Antioxidant and Anti-Inflammatory Action." *International Immunopharmacology* 20, no. 1 (May 2014): 124–130. doi:10.1016/j.intimp.2014.02.026.

Wagner, A. E., A. M. Terschluesen, and G. Rimbach. "Health Promoting Effects of Brassica-Derived Phytochemicals: From Chemopreventive and Anti-Inflammatory Activities to Epigenetic Regulation." *Oxidative Medicine and Cellular Longevity* 2013 (2013): 12 pages. Article ID 964539. http://dx.doi.org/10.1155/2013/964539.

Zimmermann, M. *Burgerstein's Handbook of Nutrition: Micronutrients in the Prevention and Therapy of Disease.* New York: Thieme, 2001.

RECIPE INDEX

INDEX

ACKNOWLEDGMENTS

I was born into a family who valued preparing our meals from scratch in spite of an active lifestyle. When I was growing up, my mom would make dinner almost every night for me and my six siblings. It would have been very expensive for us to go out to eat. Seeing her in the kitchen made me appreciate the dying art of cooking, threatened by the fast pace of our modern-day lifestyle. It is important for young children and their future health to learn this early on. I am thankful for my family teaching me that and for being receptive to the nutrition knowledge I have to share with them. They were among the first clients out of the many I have seen taking control and improving their own health.

I would not have my clinical nutrition business today if it were not for the support of my husband, Enrique. He never lets me give up and reminds me daily about the passion I have to help others get well and stay well. His encouragement keeps me going.

I also want to thank the health practitioners who have helped me regain my health and have inspired me to be the health professional I am today, specifically Dr. Stephen Dubuc and Dr. Elizabeth Miller. Without their expertise and guidance, I would not be where I am today.

Additionally, I would like to acknowledge my colleagues whom I look up to and appreciate for all their support, especially Kate Hope, who I am honored to have writing the foreword for this book.

Last, I want to thank the Callisto Media team for all their hard work. I appreciate the support they have given me to share my personal health journey and knowledge with the world.